Tell Me What to Eat As I Approach Menopause

Tell Me What to Eat As I Approach Menopause

By
Elaine Magee, MPH, RD

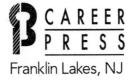
CAREER
PRESS
Franklin Lakes, NJ

Copyright © 1999 by Elaine Magee

TELL ME WHAT TO EAT AS I APPROACH MENOPAUSE
Cover design by Lu Rossman
Printed in the U.S.A. by Book-mart Press

To order this title, please call toll-free 1-800-CAREER-1 (NJ and Canada: 201-848-0310) to order using VISA or MasterCard, or for further information on books from Career Press.

The Career Press, Inc., 3 Tice Road, PO Box 687, Franklin Lakes, NJ 07417

Library of Congress Cataloging-in-Publication Data

Magee, Elaine.
Tell me what to eat as I approach menopause / by Elaine Magee.
    p. cm.
    Includes index.
    ISBN 1-56414-425-9
    1. Menopause—Nutritional aspects. 2. Menopause—Complications. Diet therapy Recipes. 3. Menopause Popular works.
4. Perimenopause
Popular works.   I. Title.
RG186.M24   1999
618.1'75—dc21   99-16766

Table of Contents

Introduction

I'm approaching 40 and I have to admit, I am afraid of a few things regarding my health. I'm afraid of cancer in any shape or form (my mother is a six-year breast cancer survivor), of being told I have developed diabetes (my father has had Type 2 diabetes for almost 20 years), of putting on even more extra pounds than I already have, oh yeah—and that little thing called menopause.

If you are about where I am in my life, or in your 40s or early 50s, you are bound to have a lot of questions and concerns about menopause. The first chapter in this book addresses many questions women have about menopause in general. The rest of the book helps you manage menopause and reduce the risk of chronic disease through one area of your life that you can do something about—an area that strongly influences your health—diet.

The 10 most common symptoms of perimenopause and what you can do to minimize them are covered in

Chapter 2. The most common questions about food and nutrition that women have during and after peri-menopause are answered in Chapter 3. The 10 Food Steps to Freedom (of perimenopause and the chronic disease risk that escalates after menopause) are described for you in Chapter 4, which basically tell you which foods to choose and which foods to lose.

The remaining chapters give you the necessary tools to take those 10 Food Steps to Freedom in comfort and style. We give you the recipes you can't live without in Chapter 5. We tell you how to navigate the supermarket and find the foods and products that are going to make your life more comfortable and healthful in Chapter 6. And we give you suggestions to make restaurant dining work in your favor in Chapter 7. Just to make sure every-thing makes sense, we will walk you through some diet makeovers of women approaching or in the middle of menopause. We will talk about specific things they can do to improve their disease risks and make themselves more comfortable for the duration.

I personally see menopause as the second "rite of pas-sage" for women—the first being childbirth. Well, I made it through the first passage—twice. I can make it through this one. Almost every postmenopausal woman has a story to tell, most based in humor, a few in horror. Here's hop-ing for humor. This was a perfect time for me to write and research this book because I am about to be this book's target audience. I had many of the questions and con-cerns that you probably have. I even spoke with a lot of women who were in the thick of it, just to make sure I hadn't missed anything. I feel a lot better now about what was formerly the unknown—perimenopause. I hope you will, too, after reading this book.

 _Chapter 1_

Everything You Ever Wanted to Ask Your Practitioner About Perimenopause

E very time you have an appointment to see your doctor or nurse practitioner you might get a golden 20 minutes alone with him or her (if you're lucky.) This doesn't leave much time to ask all the little questions you might have about what you are presently experiencing in perimenopause or what to expect after menopause.

It helps to write down your questions before you visit with your practitioner. Even if you are certain you will not forget to ask your questions, you will. I know I do. The appointment usually goes like this: You fill out some forms and hand over your medical cards, then you have a physical exam or tests that need to be done, and then you meet with your practitioner who gives you a host of information, depending on the results of your various tests. And somehow in this whirlwind of medical transactions, you inevitably end up walking out with your questions unasked and unanswered.

This chapter will answer, I hope, most of the questions you might have about perimenopause and menopause.

(The most common food and diet-related questions can be found in Chapter 3.)

Q **What does the term "menopause" refer to?**

Menopause is the permanent, natural end of ovulation (producing eggs) and menstruation. Technically, "menopause" is just one day—the day when you have not had a period for 12 consecutive months. So, basically, after this magical day, a women is considered to be "past" menopause or "postmenopausal."

Q **What does perimenopause mean?**

Perimenopause, which translates to "around" menopause or "being in" menopause, is the period of about six years before menopause (or when women are still consecutively having their period—before they haven't had their period for 12 consecutive months) and the year after menopause. During perimenopause, women's bodies are in transition. The body is starting to make the switch between being fertile and having periods to not being fertile and not having periods. Perimenopause can last about six years or more, but every woman's experience is different.

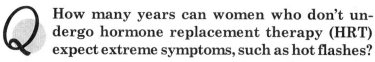

How many years can women who don't undergo hormone replacement therapy (HRT) expect extreme symptoms, such as hot flashes?

It varies from woman to woman. (I'll give you fair warning: You are going to hear this answer a lot.) With regard to hot flashes, some women have none while, on the other extreme, some women have hot flashes for five to six years. Most women, however, fall somewhere in-between (around two to three years.)

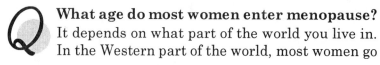

What age do most women enter menopause?

It depends on what part of the world you live in. In the Western part of the world, most women go through "natural menopause" (not caused by medical intervention) between the ages of 45 and 55 (on average at around 51). There are some early birds—women who go through menopause in their 40s and even in their 30s—and a few "late birds" who go through menopause in their 60s.

Q Are there indications of when I might go through menopause?

Start by asking your mother and older sisters. Our genetics does help determine at what age we go through menopause. Smoking is the other determinant. Smokers, and even ex-smokers, can reach menopause two or more years early. What if you started your period at an early age? The new consensus is that age of first period does *not* correlate with a woman's age at menopause.

Q Why does it seem particularly difficult for women experiencing surgical menopause or induced menopause?

[Induced menopause is immediate menopause caused by a medical intervention that removes or damages the ovaries.]

Women who have their ovaries removed really skip the whole "transition" part, or perimenopause. They instead experience immediate menopause. To put it mildly, they go through a dramatic shift in hormone levels and tend to experience much more severe symptoms—namely severe hot flashes.

In these situations, women are experiencing menopause earlier than they normally would have. Therefore, they are at greater risk of heart disease and osteoporosis because they lack the protective effects of longer estrogen treatments. When it is known in advance that a woman will have her ovaries removed, many practitioners will start estrogen therapy before surgery.

Q **What are the first signs of perimenopause?**
Most women first notice changes in their period
(see the list below) or missed periods. But women
around that golden age of perimenopause should be on
the lookout for a few other common first symptoms. Some
women, one day, might suddenly have a hot flash while
others might have a bout of night sweats. The next
perimenopause symptom may be a bit more difficult to
recognize—increased irritability as part of your premenstrual syndrome (PMS). You may experience PMS irritability when you never had before. Believe it or not, often
the number-one perimenopausal complaint of women to
their practitioners is irritability. Normal changes in your
period during perimenopause include:

- Your menstrual cycle is shorter than 28 days (for
  most women it may change to a 21 to 25 day cycle).
- Skipped periods.
- Lighter or heavier bleeding (let's hope for the
  former).
- Shorter or longer periods.

F.Y.I. *Iron supplements may be in order*

If you are one of those unlucky women who is experiencing heavy bleeding or more frequent periods
during perimenopause, you might need to take an iron
supplement to help prevent anemia. With the extra
loss of blood, you are losing extra iron as well. Your
body must make new blood to help replace the continued loss, and making new blood requires a good supply of iron. Many women don't get enough iron normally, and this extra bleeding really puts them at an
added risk of becoming anemic. Ask your practitioner
what he or she recommends.

The changes during perimenopause, although considered normal, are a reminder that you should get a medical examination immediately. These same symptoms could be caused by something not-so-normal (such as fibroids tumors, thyroid disorders, cancer or other serious disease, and even pregnancy) that needs to be treated immediately. Contact your practitioner particularly if you notice very heavy periods, often with clots of blood; periods that last two or more days longer than usual; spotting between periods; or bleeding after intercourse.

 Many friends and family members have had problems with fibroid tumors. Can you tell me more about them?

These benign growths are more common than you think—occurring in between one in three and one in four women over the age of 35. (African-American women are even more likely to have them.) I can personally attest to this statistic. I had a large fibroid removed, along with my uterus, when I was 37. I had never before had problems with fibroids. And then suddenly, only six months after my annual gynecological exam, which I passed with flying colors, I felt a mass about 7 inches long and 4 inches wide on the outside of what ended up being my uterus.

I started feeling around my lower abdomen because I had just had an unusually heavy and painful period. I wasn't sure what I was looking for really. The thought of a fibroid never even occurred to me. The only symptoms I had before this notably "unusual" period was a few sharp pains in my side a couple of months before, and unusually overactive intestinal and stomach discomfort (particularly in the morning) for a couple of months. It turned out that this fibroid was actually pressing up against my stomach, which was causing some of the stomach discomfort.

Most fibroids exist without any symptoms, but some cause symptoms ranging from heavier bleeding during your period or more frequent periods, to back pain, abnormal menstrual pain and cramps, discomfort during intercourse, and problems urinating or moving one's bowels. Sometimes, if fibroids are too big to be removed vaginally, they are taken via a lower abdominal incision (similar to a Cesarean-section cut). Sometimes the uterus is taken along with the fibroid if the woman is ready to retire her womb. It is difficult to get all the fibroid tissue and therefore the fibroids often come back within a year or two—sometimes just as big.

The North American Menopause Society estimates that 30 percent of all hysterectomies in the United States are performed to remove fibroids. It is important to keep in mind that even if just the uterus is removed (and the ovaries are left to do their important hormonal job), there is some evidence that a hysterectomy can sometimes bring on natural menopause a few years earlier than it would have been. Women who have only their ovaries will still go through perimenopause but won't experience some of the symptoms typical of normal perimenopause (such as irregular bleeding) because of the lack of a uterus.

If you have a fibroid that your practitioner is keeping an eye on, it is very important to remember that sometimes the estrogen in HRT can stimulate fibroid growth. After menopause, fibroids do tend to shrink or disappear.

Q When can I stop worrying about pregnancy?

Pregnancy remains possible until you've missed 12 consecutive periods (the point at which menopause is reached). Taking HRT (estrogen and progestogen) for menopausal symptoms does not protect you against pregnancy because the doses are usually much lower than oral contraceptives. Work with your practitioner to decide what birth control method will be most comfortable for you during this transitional time.

Q **Does menopause cause clinical depression?**
Recent studies have shown that menopause does not cause clinical depression. Menopause and depression can, of course, happen at the same time, but are separate conditions.

If you have had a previous episode (or a family history) of clinical depression, or if you are managing multiple health problems with assorted other stresses, you may be at increased risk for depression. Talk with your practitioner about what you can put into place in terms of support, therapy, and the like to maintain your mental health during this physically challenging time of your life.

Q **Will hormone therapy help my moodiness?**
Unfortunately not. In rare cases, the estrogen in hormone therapy can make matters worse in some women who are already clinically depressed. I'm afraid to say that the progestin (a synthetic progestogen) often included in hormone therapy isn't much help either. One of the common side effects to synthetic progestin is alterations in mood. You are more likely to experience this side effect if, during your younger years, mood changes were a common PMS symptom. But help is on the way— this tends to be less of a problem with women who use the newer micronised progesterone.

Q **What is the difference between estrogen replacement therapy and hormone replacement therapy?**
Most hormone replacement regimens contain a combination of the hormones estrogen and progesterone. The

combination treatment is called HRT (hormone replace-ment therapy) while ERT (estrogen replacement therapy) refers to the treatment of just the hormone estrogen. ERT is typically given to women who no longer have their uterus because ERT increases the risk of uterine cancer.

Recent literature shows that adding progesterone to your hormone therapy does not seem to lower the estro-gen protection of the bones and heart.

Q Is there a difference to using HRT with natural progesterone vs. synthetic progestin?

Fluid retention, headache, breast tenderness, and moodiness are the four possible side effects associ-ated with progestin as part of HRT. Using "natural" or micronised (pulverised into particles only a few micra in size) progesterone seems to be tolerated better, caus-ing fewer side effects. There may also be another advan-tage to taking natural progesterone over the synthetic version: heart disease prevention. Although synthetic progestin can lower the "good cholesterol" (HDLs) that taking estrogen alone can increase, natural progester-one doesn't seem to have this unwanted HDL lowering effect.

Q What are the risks and benefits of HRT?

Before we get into the pluses and minus of HRT, let me just say that when it comes to HRT, there is no right or wrong answer. Each woman has to make the decision (with her practitioner) to use or not use hor-mones based on her personal risk profile for osteoporosis, heart disease, cancer, and her perimenopause symptoms. A woman may even change her decision depending on whether she's dealing with active perimenopause symp-toms or if she is postmenopausal and concerned about chronic disease risk.

Some women have found great relief with HRT, while others have tried it and decided to go off it because the side effects for their particular body were just too unpleasant. Each woman's decision to use hormones and experience with HRT will be different. But information is power. The more information you have about your personal risk for chronic disease and what to expect with HRT, the more likely it is that you will make a decision you can live with.

HRT helps protect against osteoporosis, lower the risk of heart disease, and alleviate menopausal symptoms. That's the good news. However, along with the many benefits of HRT comes a short list of rather unpleasant side effects. There are still some questions about whether hormone replacement therapy increases the risk of certain cancers (although recent studies show that the risk is very small).

There are really only two main reasons to decide not to take hormones. The first are the unpleasant side effects:

- PMS symptoms.
- Bloating (fluid retention).
- Weight gain.
- Breast tenderness.
- Headaches.
- Nausea.
- The likely return of menstrual bleeding.

(**Note:** Women on ERT versus HRT tend to experience these side effects *less* often.)

These side effects are not to be underestimated. About 50 percent of women who are prescribed HRT stopped taking their hormones after one year, mainly because of the unpleasant side effects. I personally know several women who chose to stop taking HRT because of debilitating headaches and because they didn't like the way it made them feel.

The other main reason people think twice before taking hormones is probably one of the hottest issues debated during the past 10 years: the question of whether ERT and HRT increase the risk of certain cancers (namely uterine and breast cancer). We have known for years that when estrogen therapy is taken alone, there is most definitely an increased risk of uterine cancer. So if a woman does *not* have her uterus (because of a hysterectomy), ERT may still be given. But if a woman has her uterus, HRT is often given because the progesterone helps eliminate this increased risk of uterine cancer.

But what about the risk of other cancers? The current thinking is that estrogen does not cause new tumors to develop, but may promote the growth of existing tumors. So if you are considering hormone replacement therapy, it makes sense to have a mammogram and complete physical exam to check for any existing tumors.

Following is what we know so far about hormone therapy and breast cancer:

- Some researchers have observed up to 40 percent increase in breast cancer risk when ERT is taken for long periods of time (up to 15 years.) What about HRT? Some scientists believe when progestogen or testosterone is added to estrogen therapy, the risk of breast cancer is increased further.

- The risk of breast cancer increases as women get older. The majority of breast cancer cases occur in women older than age 50.

- Many women who develop breast cancer have no known risk factors other than growing older. Conversely, many women with known risk factors do not get breast cancer at all.

Your choice of hormone use depends on what your personal health needs are. Keep in mind that the women most at risk for osteoporosis and heart disease will reap the most benefits from HRT.

Who should *not* take hormones?

You should *absolutely not* opt for hormone therapy (ERT or HRT) if you:

- currently have or recently had uterine cancer.
- currently have or recently had an estrogen-sensitive breast cancer or tumor.
- have active liver disease.
- have active thrombophlebitis (inflammation of a vein in conjunction with the formation of a clot; usually occurs in a leg) or thromboembolism (the blocking of a blood vessel by a blood clot that has broken off from where it was formed).
- have vaginal bleeding of unknown cause.

You should *probably not* go on hormone replacement therapy (ERT or HRT) if you have:

- a history of uterine cancer.
- large uterine fibroids.
- endometriosis.
- a history of breast cancer.
- a history of thrombophlebitis or thromboembolism.
- a history of stroke or transient ischemic attack (temporary interference with blood supply to the brain).
- a history of recent heart attack.
- hypertension aggravated by estrogen.
- migraine headaches aggravated by estrogen.
- pancreatic disease.
- gallbladder disease.
- a history of liver disease.

You might also want to discuss hormone therapy (ERT or HRT) carefully with your practitioner if you have one or more of the following:

- a family history of estrogen-dependent cancers of the breast, uterus, or ovaries.
- elevated blood lipids (hyperlipidemia, high serum cholesterol), because the progesterone may undesirably alter your blood lipids.
- severe high blood pressure.
- severe varicose veins, because it increases the risk of clots.
- a combination of health concerns, such as obesity, high blood pressure, smoking, varicose veins.
- diabetes.
- immune system disorders.
- kidney disease.
- multiple sclerosis.
- epilepsy.
- Dublin-Johnson syndrome (unexplainable jaundice).

Q A question you may not ask, but you need to know about...
Postmenopausal women without adequate estrogen levels may have an increased risk for sexually transmitted diseases (STDs). The vaginal tissue in menopausal women becomes increasingly more delicate and is more prone to small tears and cuts during intercourse, which can make infection even more likely.

The aftermath of menopause

Okay. So you've made it through the hot flashes, night sweats, and surprise periods. Maybe you have officially celebrated the end of menstruation. In that case, you may have questions about what to expect in your postmenopausal years including questions about risks for certain diseases, namely heart disease and osteoporosis. Here are a few.

Q **How does menopause affect blood pressure and cholesterol?**

Postmenopausal women are at greater risk of high blood pressure—about half of women beyond age 55 have high blood pressure. (Blood pressure is often regarded as high when your reading is greater than 140/90 mm Hg.) Even mild elevations of blood pressure can double your risk of stroke. The scariest thing about high blood pressure is that there are usually no symptoms—nada—none. That's why high blood pressure is nicknamed "the silent killer." You could have raging high blood pressure and you won't feel much different. So it is absolutely essential to have your blood pressure taken regularly.

Keeping an eye on our blood values of serum cholesterol and triglycerides helps give us an idea of what's going on inside our heart and arteries. Our blood levels of certain lipids can either encourage or discourage fatty plaque to build up in our arterial walls. When you have your blood lipids tested, make sure that the low density lipoprotein (LDL or "bad cholesterol") levels are tested along with the high density lipoproteins (HDL or "good cholesterol"). Another lipid level that is usually tested for is triglycerides. The normal, healthy range is 85 to 200 mg/dL. If you have elevated triglycerides, in addition to exercising, limiting alcohol, maintaining a healthy weight, and not smoking, there are certain things you can do to help lower them. They include making sure your diet contains some omega-3 fatty acids and monounsaturated fats.

There are several very promising over-the-counter products that may help reduce the risk of heart disease currently under investigation—vitamin E, folic acid (folate), soy foods, and daily aspirin intake.

 If I have a family history of heart disease (or other key risk factors) should I consider taking hormone replacement therapy?

When making the decision for or against taking hormones, this is certainly one of the items to consider, along with the severity of your perimenopause symptoms and your personal risk for osteoporosis or estrogen-dependent cancers.

It is a fact that after menopause when your estrogen levels have plummeted, your risk for heart disease does increase. This puts the women who experienced premature menopause (natural or induced) at an even greater risk. ERT may reduce the risk of heart disease by as much as 50 percent (studies are being conducted to provide more information on the actual percentage risk reduction). Estrogen mainly helps by raising HDL ("good cholesterol") and by lowering LDL ("bad cholesterol"). It reduces the rate of growth of fatty deposits in blood vessels and helps keep blood vessels open. But here's something you should know: If you have established heart disease and you start hormone therapy using a continuous, combined regimen of estrogen plus progestogen, you do not receive protection against heart disease.

You are at risk for cardiovascular disease if you have the following (the more factors you have, the higher your risk):

_____ I smoke.

_____ My total serum cholesterol is more than 200 mg/dL.

_____ My LDL ("bad cholesterol") is more than 130 mg/dL.

_____ My serum triglycerides are more than 200 mg/dL.

_____ My HDL ("good cholesterol") is less than 35 mg/dL.

____ My ratio of total serum cholesterol to HDL cholesterol is more than 4.5:1 (to calculate this, divide
your total cholesterol by your HDLs).

____ I have high blood pressure.

____ I am diabetic.

____ I have a family history of premature heart disease
(heart disease before age 55 in one of your parents).

Q **What should I know about osteoporosis?**
In osteoporosis, the protein matrix of bone and
mineral deposits is gradually lost, decreasing the
total amount of bone and weakening the skeleton, making the bones more susceptible to fractures (particularly
the hip, spine, and wrist bones).

Estrogen helps maintain bone density. So, as estrogen levels naturally decline, bone loss increases. Until
around age 33, your body builds your bones. By the time
menopause rolls around, your total bone mass has already
started to gradually decline. But there is something you
can do: You can preserve the bone mass you currently
have. About one-third of postmenopausal women have or
will have osteoporosis. But osteoporosis is preventable
and treatable in most women.

There are some easy, painless tests you can take so
your practitioner can take a good look at your bone density and determine if you are likely to have a problem
down the line. It is very important to find bone-density
problems early so treatments can begin early.

Genetics is certainly one factor determining your like-
lihood of getting osteoporosis. Your own lifestyle choices,
however, also come into play. Some bone metabolism experts believe that half of your bone loss after age 30 is
influenced by lifestyle factors, such as alcohol use (heavy
alcohol intake increases your risk), exercise habits
(weight-bearing exercise especially decreases your risk),

and a healthy diet (see Chapter 3 for more on ways to decrease your risk through the foods you choose).

Experts believe that ERT (with proper diet and lifestyle choices) is the best way to prevent osteoporosis, reducing spine, hip, and wrist fractures by 50 to 75 percent when taken for many years. If you are indeed at high risk for osteoporosis, the time may be now for estrogen therapy. It makes sense that estrogen therapy would reduce the most bone loss (and have the biggest benefit) if taken when the rate of bone loss is greatest—during the five to 10 years following menopause. However, the benefits continue only as long as the estrogen is taken. Therefore, once you start, you can't really stop.

You are at risk for osteoporosis if you have the following (the more factors you have the higher your risk):

_____ I smoke.

_____ I am Caucasian.

_____ I am underweight for my height.

_____ I am fair-skinned.

_____ My mother or grandmother (or other female blood relatives) grew stooped with age or had osteoporosis.

_____ I drink more than three servings of soda (carbonated beverages containing phosphoric acid, which contains phosphorus, compete with calcium for absorption in the intestines).

_____ I take thyroid supplements.

_____ I have chronic digestion problems.

This chapter was written thanks to interviews with The North American Menopause Society (NAMS)* and one of my favorite nurse practitioners, Patricia Geraghty FNP, MSN (who was also my Lamaze instructor many years ago). You can reach the NAMS at the following address:

The North American Menopause Society
P.O. Box 94527
Cleveland, OH 44101
216-844-8748 (or 800-774-5342)
www.menopause.org

 _Chapter 2_

The Top 9 Symptoms of Perimenopause...and How to Eat Your Way Around Them

E very woman experiences a different perimenopause. Most women have some hot
flashes, some irritability, and a smaller number
battle headaches, nausea, or night sweats. Whatever your
symptoms, the following common-sense food strategies
might just help make your perimenopause a little more
comfortable.

Charting your course through perimenopause using
only food strategies may be rather rough waters. The
trouble is that treating perimenopause symptoms is like
hitting a moving target. What works for one woman may
not work for another, and what works for you now may
not work as well a year from now. In addition, what _didn't_
work earlier for perimenopausal symptoms may help you
later on. It is, for many, a trial and error situation that
continues for several years, where you are constantly fir-
ing away at the various discomforts that pop up using
the food and herb arsenal of the modern kitchen.

The truth is that many of the diet suggestions in this chapter are things we should all be doing anyway—many years before menopause. But for whatever reason, many of us haven't quite gotten in the habit of eating more fruits and vegetables, for example, even though we know they are good for us. In perimenopause, many women suddenly find themselves motivated to make these changes. Is it because we are uncomfortable and desperately want relief? Is it because we are faced with sobering statistics about increased risk for heart disease? Is menopause the milestone that, overnight, makes us feel a whole lot more mortal? Is it that we are finally at a time in our lives when we have the freedom to focus on our own health? If perimenopause is what finally motivates someone to make important changes in her diet and lifestyle, terrific! Whatever works.

One of our best dietary defenses during perimenopause may be a diet rich in phytoestrogens. (Phytoestrogens, estrogen-like substances found in plants, are weak forms of the estrogen our premenopausal body normally produces.) Some women have found relief with daily doses of phytoestrogen-rich foods (more on this in Chapter 4).

Keep in mind that most of the following suggestions have not had the benefit of well-designed clinical trials, so it is difficult to predict how well they will work for you. But many women are having some success with these nonhormonal remedies—especially for mild symptoms. Most of the food suggestions don't cost much, and most are healthy changes we should be making in our lives anyway.

#1 *Is it just me or are you hot, too?*

By far, the most common discomfort of perimenopause is the hot flash. Up to 80 percent of all women have hot flashes during perimenopause. My guess is, it is one of those things you have to experience yourself to truly know what it feels like. But let me give it a try below, just so you might know what to expect should it start happening to you.

Some women may simply "get too hot" more often than before. It is also possible to have a chill without the hot flash, although it happens to very few women.

Hot flashes can go on for a few months or up to five years, although most women will flash for a couple of years. There is no way to predict how many years or months your particular hot flashes will continue.

Different things help different people

Some women say they have found relief from hot flashes by taking vitamin E supplements (400 IU per day).

F.Y.I. Anatomy of a hot flash

When estrogen levels change, usually with a sudden *decrease* in estrogen, a change in the body's circulation results.

It starts in the brain in the area that regulates body temperature. Your face and/or upper body will suddenly feel warm. This will lead to blushing, and sometimes rapid and profuse sweating. Then your heart will beat faster. For the grand finale, you may feel a cold chill.

A hot flash can last less than one minute or up to five or 10 minutes. A hot flash can even occur in a series (a few minutes apart.) Hot flashes usually have a consistent pattern, but alas, each woman's pattern is unique to her. Hot flashes can be mild to severe, ranging from a little embarrassing or annoying to completely debilitating.

Some say eating or drinking two servings of soy a day keeps the hot flashes away. The theory on the benefits of soy comes almost directly from the fact that hot flashes in Asian women, who consume soy on a daily basis, are almost nonexistent.

Following are foods that offer many women relief:

- A daily serving of **soy** (such as soy milk, tofu, tempeh, miso).

- In addition to or other than soy, **phytoestrogen-rich foods** (such as papaya, peas, beans, and lentils). See Chapter 4 for a complete list.

Following are supplements that seem to offer some women relief:

- **Vitamin E** supplements of about 400 IU daily may help some women relieve more moderate hot flashes (although the evidence for this is mostly anecdotal). A supplement is the only way to go here, because it is practically impossible to reach even 50 IUs of vitamin E with food. Take this fat-soluble vitamin with a meal or snack that contains some fats for easier digestion.

  Vitamin E supplements aren't a bad idea even if you're not having hot flashes but menopause is knocking at your door. There is some evidence that suggests that this amount of vitamin E supplementation helps your immune system and could promote a better lipid profile, which in turn helps prevent cardiovascular disease. There is no evidence at this time of toxic effects at this level of supplementation.

- **Vitamin C** supplements of 1,000 milligrams per day have also been listed as potentially helpful to some women.

- **Flaxseed** is actually a seed, but because you take it more as a supplement, it is best listed here. Flaxseed contributes quite a few powerful substances to our everyday diet. In the case of hot flashes, however, it is a super rich source of the phytoestrogen *lignin*. Generally one to two teaspoons of ground flaxseed per day seems to be very helpful to some women. (Grind a week's suppy at a time and keep it refrigerated).

Give it time

In today's world, we are used to instant gratification. Unfortunately, discovering whether certain diet therapies are truly helping requires time and patience. For vitamin E supplements, it may take two to six weeks before you see any results. For soy foods, it may be four to six weeks before they start to take effect.

Sometimes it isn't what you add, but what you take away, that helps

Some women find that avoiding certain foods and beverages works best for them. As devastating as this may sound, that cup or two of java you have every morning may be triggering some of your hot flashes. What's more, there are several other favorites that are considered to be hot flash "trigger foods."

Basically, the big three to avoid are hot and spicy foods, caffeine, and alcohol. You may also find that hot drinks trigger hot flashes. You might even find that you need to avoid these triggers at certain times of the day.

When you have a hot flash, consider whether you had one of the trigger foods minutes or a few hours before the hot flash. Hot and spicy foods and hot drinks tend to have an instantaneous effect on hot flashes (within minutes), while alcohol and caffeine can have an effect 30 minutes to two to four hours later. Try avoiding these triggers to see whether your hot flashes lessen.

Leave the large meals to the men

Large meals can also increase your body temperature. When you eat a large meal, especially one high in fat, there is a lot of digesting and metabolizing going on—which generates extra heat. It is easier to feel faint and sluggish after a large meal as well because a lot of blood is diverted to the stomach, leaving less blood to circulate through the rest of your body, part of which brings oxygen to the brain.

Keep your cool in more ways than one

Not only are there hot flash trigger foods, there are hot flash trigger situations. Emotionally upsetting and stressful situations, high-temperature situations (in and outdoors), and poorly ventilated rooms can help trigger hot flashes, too. Many women find relief by dressing in layers, so they can easily peel off a layer or two when needed to cool down during the day. You might even try using a small fan at work. If possible, keep a glass of ice chips near or desk while at work or your bed at home and start sucking on ice at the first sign of a hot flash or night sweat.

"Taking a cold shower" can take on a whole new meaning in perimenopause. Some women find that if they take a cool 20-minute bath or cold shower in the morning keeps them virtually flush-free throughout the day. This tip might be most practical during the warmer summer months.

Just breathe

Deep breathing can even help some women through their hot flashes. Take deep, slow breaths that start in your abdomen: Take five seconds to breathe in the air and five seconds to breathe it out—about six to eight breaths per minute. You can practice this breathing a couple of times a day and then use it whenever a hot flash starts.

Some women get the edge on hot flashes by using imagery. When they feel a hot flash coming on, they immediately start imagining a much "cooler" place. For example, let your mind wander to the cool ocean, feel the breeze on your face as you splash about in the icy water. You could imagine being in the shade at the bottom of an icy waterfall or sitting on the cool moss as you dip your toes into the icy water. Feel the cool mist of the waterfall refresh your body as it kissees your face. Get the idea?

Reducing stress is a good idea for all-around good health, but is especially helpful during perimenopause. Do whatever you feel comfortable with to reduce the stress in your life. Just exercising regularly really helps some women reduce stress. Some women meditate or take a yoga class while others find regular massages and relaxing baths to be helpful. (Sign me up for the regular massages anytime!)

#2 Who poured a bucket of water over me?

When hot flashes hit during sleeptime leaving you in a puddle of perspiration, they are called "night sweats." The good news is that all the hot flash prevention suggestions above would also help prevent night sweats.

The trouble with night sweats is, even if they don't wake you up, they could still be disturbing your much needed rest. If night sweats are troubling you, it is particularly important to avoid those hot flash trigger foods before bedtime. And if you aren't in a regular exercise program already, this is just yet another reason to start: Regular exercise (pick something you actually *like* to do) encourages deeper, more productive sleep.

Because a "warm environment" is also considered to be a hot flash trigger, sleep in something thin and made of cotton, keep the bedroom on the cool side, and perhaps even point a fan directly at your side of the bed. You won't have to wait weeks to know if this is working. You should know within a few days!

#3 Dealing with insomnia

Insomnia during perimenopause is different than normal insomnia when you can't *fall* asleep. With perimenopausal insomnia, you get to sleep just fine, but you wake up in the middle of the night and cannot get back to sleep (secondary insomnia). If this has happened to you, you know how frustrating it is! You might find that your insomnia follows a pattern around your menstrual (hormonal) cycle. The insomnia tends to be more frequent during the week before menstruation and around ovulation (the middle of your cycle).

So what are your options? Over-the-counter sleep medications are probably not going to help women in the midst of perimenopausal insomnia. There are a few good food and lifestyle tricks you can try first. Then, if all else fails, see your practitioner to discuss your pharmaceutical or hormonal options. You definitely do not want to go through your perimenopausal years walking around like a zombie with jet lag.

The first thing you will want to do is avoid stimulants such as caffeine, especially after 5 or 6 p.m. If that doesn't work, you should stop consuming caffeine even earlier in the day (around 2 p.m.) to see if that helps. Caffeine can be found in coffee, tea, certain soft drinks, and to a lesser degree in chocolate. Also check for caffeine in any prescriptions and over-the-counter drugs.

Avoid drinking alcohol late at night, too. Many women can still enjoy a glass of wine with dinner (as long as it isn't a late dinner). Alcohol fools you by making you think you're sleepy, but it doesn't help you get restful sleep. It disturbs your deep-sleep phases and wakes you up several times during the night. Following are a few other things you can eat or drink to try and induce quality sleep.

Carbo-load in the evening

High carbohydrate meals tend to induce sleep better than high-protein meals. It is suspected that the amino acid in many high carbohydrate foods—tryptophan—is converted in the brain to serotonin, which is a sleep-inducing neurotransmitter. A high carbo meal may also produce more heat as a by-product of digestion and metabolism, which in turn helps encourage sleepiness. Although we don't know why or how, scientists have observed that high carbo meals also increase the duration of total sleep by lengthening some of the individual sleep stages.

What about the warm milk old wives tale?

It doesn't appear that warm milk has the amount of chemicals needed to truly "chemically" induce sleep, but psychologically, warm milk relaxes us by reminding many of us of comforting moments in our past.

Don't go to bed angry—or hungry!

Strong hunger can wake you up from a sound sleep. Of course, it isn't good to go to sleep really full either. You might find light hunger is fine or that being somewhere in between hungry and comfortably full works best. If you're still hungry just before bed, but don't want to eat another meal, you might want to try having a carbohydrate-rich snack such as fruit, breakfast cereal, or a slice or two of bread.

Exercise does more than build strong bodies—it builds better sleep

Regular exercise (especially in the late afternoon or early morning hours) promotes deeper stages of sleep. But exercising late at night could work against you. Often, exercising in the evening will give you a burst of post-exercise energy. There are times when you might want this late night burst of energy, but if you don't want it to interfere with your normal sleep schedule, try not to exercise much later than 6 or 7 p.m.

Bedtime teas and potions

For hundreds of years, our ancestors have used herbs to help them sleep. One of the oldest herbal remedies known for its sedative and sleep-inducing effects is now called Valerian (valeriana officinalis). It comes most often in the form of tea and is considered very safe.

#4 More frequent sex: The solution to vaginal dryness

There's no pretty way to say this: Many women notice a dryness, irritation, and/or itching in and around their vulva and vagina during perimenopause. Probably most unsettling though is that many women also experience discomfort during intercourse.

The natural decreases in estrogen seem to encourage this thinning and drying of the vulvavaginal tissue, which then make the tissue more likely to be irritated and injured during intercourse or even a pelvic examination. The lower estrogen levels also tend to make the vaginal area less acidic (encouraging bacteria growth).

These changes can range from being a slight pain, literally, to being extremely disturbing. In any case, you will want your doctor or nurse practitioner to make sure your discomfort is not being caused by something non-menopausal (bacterial infection, sexually transmitted disease, etc...) that needs a specific treatment.

You are more at risk for these vaginal changes if you:

- aren't experiencing regular sexual stimulation of the vagina.
- experience premature menopause.
- have a history of temporary amenorrhea (stopping of periods) resulting from over exercising, dieting, or extreme emotional distress.

There are a few things you can do to help maintain your vaginal tissue and decrease any potential problems and discomfort. Believe it or not, regular sexual activity actually helps the situation. There are even vaginal creams and lubricants specifically indicated for use in the vagina Applying vitamin E oil directly to the irritated vaginal tissue may help. A naturopathic tri-estrogen cream is available in some pharmacies. It is not a good idea, however, to apply vaginal creams containing phytoestrogens or any other hormones right before intercourse; you don't want these substances passed onto your partner. A new vaginal ring that contains estrogen is also available.

There are also some dietary measures you can take to make yourself more comfortable:

- Try eating foods that are high in phytoestrogens (plant-based forms of weak estrogens) if you cannot or wish not to use prescription-strength estrogen.

- Soy foods offer some improvement in vaginal discomfort for some women (although it might not be noticed for three to six weeks).

- Acidophilus (lactobacillus acidophilus cultures) may help to maintain the vaginal pH that starts changing with age. A dose of 460 milligrams a day supplies the amount of acidophilus in eight cups of yogurt.

- Chasteberry, taken in tea, is said to revitalize vaginal tissue.

#5 A better bladder or bust

The burn, the constant trips to the toilet, the never-ending pressure causing you discomfort or pain. If you are the one to four or five women who have occasional urinary tract infections (UTI), you know the drill. I remember being in the emergency room in the middle of the night and turning in a pink urine sample. After that night, I vowed, "as God is my witness, I will never be caught without bladder-specific antibiotics again." When it comes to UTIs, I can honestly say I know your pain.

In the throws of perimenopause and thereafter, many women begin to have problems with their bladder and urinary tract. What kind of problems? They basically fall in the "use it" or "lose it" categories. Some women have problems "using" it (their bladder):

- Urinating more often.
- Having a sudden sense of urgency, but without the full bladder to go with it.
- Needing to urinate throughout the night, and thus disturbing your desperately-needed sleep time.
- Experiencing pain during urination.

And some women have problems "losing" it (urine). If you are approaching menopause, you might have already noticed that a little urine sometimes leaks out at the most inopportune times. It might happen when you sneeze or cough, laugh or lift something.

What's going on? The lining of the urethra (outlet for the bladder) can start to thin, and the surrounding pelvic muscles can start to weaken. This combination causes the above situations to occur—courtesy of, in part, decreasing levels of estrogen. If you are the one in four women who tend to have occasional bladder infections and UTIs, leakage and urinary incontinence (which I will discuss later) are just that much more likely. So it behooves us to do whatever we can with our diet and lifestyle to keep the bladder happy.

The first thing we can do is avoid anything that irritates the bladder. This might not be as easy as it sounds because it means avoiding (or limiting) smoking, alcohol, and caffeine. Alcohol and caffeine are natural diuretics, which means they stimulate the bladder to release urine, encouraging dehydration. The more dehydrated your body is, the more concentrated your urine (because there isn't enough water in the body to go around). The more concentrated the urine, the harder it is on the bladder and the more likely bacteria is to cause a problem. Carbonated beverages (with or without caffeine) are also thought to irritate the bladder. Some women also find that oxalic acid (found in both tea and tomatoes) and vitamin C supplements irritate their bladder and vulvavaginal tissue.

You can also keep your bladder happy and healthy by helping prevent UTIs. You can do this by drinking about 10 ounces of cranberry juice a day (or eating a bowl of blueberries in their stead). We've known that cranberry juice can help keep infections away, but scientists weren't sure exactly why this is. Cranberries and blueberries reportedly contain condensed tannins called proanthocyanidins that prevent infection-causing *E. coli* bacteria from attaching to cells in the urinary tract. And if they can't attach, the bacteria are less likely to cause infection.

Studies have shown that you need to drink the juice for at least four weeks before you notice any "preventive" effects.

Beware, though. If a little is good, more may not be better. Too much cranberry juice is suspected to actually irritate the bladder. To avoid this, keep your cranberry juice intake to 10 ounces a day.

The worst case scenario is what is called "urinary incontinence": when leakage is severe enough to impact a person's well-being and/or hygiene. We've all seen those commercials on television featuring spry seniors telling us how protective adult undergarments have helped them. We usually think, "That's not going to happen to me" or "That's further on down the road for me." Well, you would be surprised, as I was, how close that roadblock might be. I was shocked to learn that up to about 40 percent of women between the ages of 45 and 64 suffer from urinary incontinence. It is very important that anyone experiencing incontinence have a thorough exam to determine the cause and discuss your options.

#6 Breast swelling, okay, but breast pain?

Some women have more breast pain when they're under stress, so putting your stress reduction strategies in motion may help with this symptom. You might want to try eliminating coffee (even decaffeinated) to see if this helps you.

Clinical observations and anecdotal evidence suggest that some women find relief when they take approximately 300 IU of vitamin E (in a supplement) per day.

Some women have reported relief with evening primrose oil supplements. Evening primrose oil does indeed contain gamma-linoleic acid which has been shown to have antiinflammatory and analgesic effects. The dose often used for mastalgia (severe breast pain) is 3 to 4 grams per day. The only trouble with this is that you may need to use it for three months before you feel any relief.

#7 When you really do have a headache

Changes in hormone levels (whether due to HRT or natural perimenopause) can also be a real pain for some women—headache pain that is. Besides the usual aspirin remedy, here are a couple of ways you can try to prevent the headache from starting.

- Even if your headaches aren't being triggered by the common trigger foods (alcohol in red wine—Chianti—and beer, tyramine in aged cheeses, pickled herring, and chocolate), consuming them in large quantities would certainly be adding insult to injury.

- *Gradually* decrease your caffeine consumption to avoid the most common pitfall of sudden caffeine withdrawal: headache.

Alternative therapies to the rescue

Following are descriptions of the two nutrition supplements and the two botanical medicines that have been reported to help some women prevent migraine headaches:

- **Magnesium:** 250 to 400 milligrams, three times a day.
- **Vitamin B6:** 25 milligrams three times per day
- **Ginger (Zingiber officinalis):** Candied ginger is probably the way many people will choose to get their ginger root. 500 milligrams of the candied ginger four times a day is a recommended dose. Approximately 10 grams of fresh ginger per day can also be used. This may be the way to go if you are having nausea along with your headache. Chewing on candied ginger also helps many women with nausea. There are no known contraindications for ginger root, although people with gallstones should probably not use it because ginger stimulates bowel secretions.
- **Feverfew:** Parthenolide is considered to be the primary chemical in feverfew responsible for the prevention of migraines. Some people may experience gastrointestinal disturbances the first week of use. Feverfew is not to be used during pregnancy and it should not be taken with nonsteroidal antiinflammatory drugs (NSAIDs). A 300-milligrams dose of feverfew, which should contain 250 micrograms parthenolide, can be taken three times a day when a migraine is present.

#8 Battling nauseousness

Many women think that because they didn't become nauseous during their pregnancy that they won't be nauseous during perimenopause either. Unfortunately that's not how it works. The big difference between nausea during pregnancy and nausea during perimenopause is with pregnancy, the nausea usually lasts three months. In perimenopause, it can go on for years. And in perimenopause, there isn't a pattern to the nausea, it can strike at any time of day.

When perimenopausal nausea starts to rear its ugly head, you need immediate relief. Some women also have an exaggerated gag reflex, making swallowing over-the-counter tablets and liquids difficult. Many women at the first sign of nausea, chew on some candied ginger. It can bring immediate relief. You can also try eating small, frequent meals throughout the day to avoid a "full" stomach. Avoid intake of stomach irritants such as coffee and spicy or acidic foods (tomatoes and orange juice) on an empty stomach.

#9 Who says I'm moody?

With unpredictable periods and nausea, nerve-racking hot flashes, and restless sleep, it's no wonder you're moody. When moodiness strikes, the last thing you need are substances considered to be depressants—like alcohol or caffeine. Because caffeine is a stimulant, it can bring you up with high energy, then down with low energy. So you might try to determine if caffeine is making matters worse. Another factor to mood swings may be concentrated sweets (chocolate cake, cookies and other such sweets). On an empty stomach, sweets could cause high then low blood sugar, ultimately making you feel sluggish and moody. Try eating concentrated sweets only with a meal.

One of the best things you can do to keep your mood on an even keel is to eat regular meals. Don't skip. Don't deprive yourself. If you are hungry, eat something. Try to have an even supply of balanced meals and/or snacks throughout the day.

Grumpy? Carbs to the rescue

Carbohydrates may also help you maintain a better mood. It all comes down to the powerful nerve chemical serotonin. Women who fight mild depression during or after menopause might have lower serotonin levels than other women. When serotonin levels are low, you are likely to crave sweets and/or feel grumpy. Simply speaking, when serotonin levels are boosted in the brain, so is your mood.

Carbohydrate-rich foods eaten in the nick of time can help increase serotonin levels in the brain. Make a list of some of your healthier carbohydrate-rich favorite snacks and have one as an in-between meal mood-lifter. Lowfat popcorn, bagels, cereals, soft and hard pretzels are my favorites.

Supplements and herbs that can help temper your moods

One of the herbal remedies that has shown to be helpful for depression, anxiety, and nervous restlessness that is also considered to be safe with long term use is St. John's Wort. The recommended dose is 300 milligrams three times a day. Although it is hard to be patient when you are anxious and irritable, you will probably have to wait six to eight weeks before you notice any positive effects.

The other herb that may help is Valerian, which comes most commonly as a tea (see the discussion on insomnia). Another herb, kava kava, which comes from a shrub in the South Pacific, can be a mood elevator in doses of 60 milligrams three times a day. But it doesn't have the proven long-term safety of the others and should not to be taken for more than three months without medical supervision. Speak to your practitioner before beginning these herbal remedies.

What about herbal remedies?

Some health practitioners claim that moderate hot flashes can be relieved by sipping ginseng tea. Ginseng does have a steroid-like chemical structure, suggesting that it may have an estrogen-like effect on the body. But there have been a few reports noting abnormal uterine bleeding with the use of ginseng, so consult your practitioner before trying this herbal remedy. Ginseng can also lower blood sugar and should not be used if you have high blood pressure.

Dong quai and black cohosh are two herbs you will often see associated with menopausal symptoms. Neither of these herbs have yet received FDA approval, however. The active compounds in them have not been identified and the risks and benefits of taking each of them are not yet clear. With that said, dong quai does seem to contain a natural estrogen-like substance and it may have some therapeutic effects. As it so happens, dong quai is also the only herb being studied scientifically by the United States for its effects on menopausal symptoms.

Dong quai has been touted to help reduce hot flashes, vaginal dryness, headaches, insomnia, and anxiety. It may take up to two months before you see any results. Dong quai can be taken as a tea (4 to 8 ounces a day) or 10 to 40 drops one to three times a day used in tincture form. It can produce an itchy rash in some. A warning: The dong quai from China may contain Saffrole, a known carcinogen, so your only safe bet is to buy dong quai that comes from Korea.

Although some sources have found black cohosh to be effective with hot flashes and nervous conditions associated with menopause, it shouldn't be taken for more than six months, because its long-term safety is uncertain. The trouble with this herb is that you may not feel its effects until two months after beginning taking it. Some other problems: Possible side effects in higher doses include dizziness, nausea, diarrhea, abdominal pain, headache, joint pains, and decreased heart rate; and it should not be used by anyone with heart disease.

Remember, when it comes to using herbs therapeutically (even though they have been used for centuries) they are new to traditional medicine. Talk to your practitioner about what herbs you are thinking about taking so he or she can monitor your progress and continued health.

Although herbs are natural substances, exercise caution when using them. Just because they come from nature does not mean they are harmless—many herbs have drug-like properties. Incidentally, many modern drugs we use today come from "natural" sources. Marijuana and tobacco are technically "herbs," and cocaine technically comes from a shrub native to Bolivia and Peru. Although these substances are natural, no one would call them harmless. Use caution when taking any herbs.

 *Chapter 3*

Everything You Ever Wanted to Ask a Dietitian About Menopause

Q **How can diet and foods help me if I choose to go on HRT?**

You can use your diet and the foods you eat to help minimize some of the health risks and side effects you might experience on HRT. For example, make sure you are getting plenty of antioxidant-rich and phytochemical-rich fruits and vegetables. They will help protect your body against cancer. Following the 10 Food Steps to Freedom (Chapter 4) will also help minimize your risk of disease.

Many women stop taking hormones mainly because of the side effects. Women complain of five major side effects resulting from HRT. Following is a list of the these side effects and some dietary or lifestyle suggestions for possible relief.

To relieve bloating:

- Make sure you are well hydrated; drink about eight cups of water (or other decaffeinated beverage) every day.

- Eat a fairly low-sodium diet (no more than 2,400 milligrams of sodium per day).
- Avoid caffeine and alcohol, which are diuretics (they increase the loss of urine, even if the body needs this water to remain well-hydrated). But natural, more gentle diuretics like watermelon, lemon, grapefruit juice, and cucumber might actually help in normal portions.

To relieve headaches:

- Avoid red wine and beer.
- Avoid caffeine and chocolate and tyramine in aged cheeses, Chianti wine, and pickled herring.
- If you are trying to reduce your caffeine intake, remember to taper it gradually—don't stop all of a sudden. Headache is the most common symptom of caffeine withdrawal.
- Refer back to Chapter 2 for more recommendations to lessen headache pain.

To reduce weight gain:

Weight gain is a common side effect of all forms of hormone therapy (even birth control pills). So please don't beat yourself up about it. It is obviously a good idea to keep the weight gain to a minimum though, so this might be a good time to double check a few things.

- Are you enjoying regular exercise?
- Are you eating when you are hungry and stopping when you are comfortably full? Try eating several small meals throughout the day and eating light at night. This will help increase your metabolism. Eliminating those large meals that tend to lead to lethargy and extra calories hitting the bloodstream all at once should help, too.

- Are you eating a lower-fat diet, rich in fruits and vegetables and grains, that is also delicious and satisfying?

To relieve nausea:

Nausea is one of those side effects you should most definitely talk to your practitioner about. Varying the dose or the time of day that you take the hormones may help. (For other suggestions on handling nausea, please see Chapter 2.)

To relieve breast tenderness:

- Work with your practitioner to adjust the dose of estrogen or use natural progesterone. (For other suggestions on breast pain, see Chapter 2.)

 After menopause a woman's risk of heart disease starts to equal a man's. How can I lower my risk through the foods I choose?

There's no way around it. Estrogen helps protect women from heart disease in so many different ways. It decreases bad cholesterol, while increasing good cholesterol in the blood. Estrogen also decreases levels of homocysteine, a chemical in the blood that is linked to clogged arteries. (High levels are associated with high heart disease risk.) Estrogen keeps the bad cholesterol from mixing with oxygen and becoming more likely to stick to the artery wall.

Once you pass through menopause, the benefits of estrogen pass as well. You can approach this fact of post-menopausal life in two ways: Use HRT or ERT and do everything in your power nutritionally to improve your risk factors for heart disease.

To help you picture the nonhormonal ways to reduce your coronary vascular disease risk, following is a short list of lifestyle changes with estimates of the percentage the change can reduce your risk.

Lifestyle change	Risk reduction (%)
Stop smoking	50%
Exercise regularly	45%
Achieve "ideal" body weight	45%
Take aspirin (325 mg/day)	33%
Reduce high blood pressure	2%[a]
Improve elevated blood lipids	2%[b]

[a]Two percent reduction in risk for each mmHg decrease in your blood pressure.
[b]Two percent reduction in risk for each one percent reduction in total cholesterol

By looking at the results in the table one can assume that you would want to be of a fairly normal weight, be a nonsmoker with a healthful diet, and would want to exercise regularly. (Additionally, it has been shown that cardiovascular risk lessens with prophylactic use of aspirin.) For more on what this "healthful diet" looks like (one that encourages a healthful lipid level, normal blood pressure, and body weight) see Chapter 4.

When it comes to the fats, basically we want to keep trans fatty acids, saturated fat, and omega-6 fatty acids (found in polyunsaturated fats) low, leaving monounsaturated fats and omega-3 fatty acids as our fats of choice—fats that may be beneficial for our health in reasonable, moderate amounts.

What about food cholesterol? Oh sure, it's a good idea not to go hog wild on high cholesterol foods, but if there are foods that are otherwise reasonably low in fat and contribute other beneficial substances such as monounsaturated fats or omega-3s (like shrimp and squid), then I think we can cut them a little slack. What about egg yolks, boasting around 210 milligrams a pop? In most recipes, I automatically use half of the egg yolk. It isn't necessarily because of the cholesterol, although that's part of it. Each yolk also contains 5 grams of fat. If I can cut them down a little without changing the food I'm making, then I do it, but keep in mind, egg yolks also contain some monounsaturated fat and vitamin E, so you may not want to cut them out entirely.

The next thing you need to do is call on our friends the antioxidants—daily. All the antioxidants (beta carotene and other carotenes, vitamin A, vitamin E, vitamin C, and phytochemicals such as the flavonoids) help us fight free radicals in the body, which, if not neutralized can cause all sorts of damage—from cancer to heart disease. But each antioxidant acts (on our body's behalf) in different ways, so we really need all of them. Vitamin E, for example, protects against oxidative damage to LDL (bad) cholesterol (oxidation makes LDL particles harmful), it reduces the stickiness of the platelets (a component in the blood), thins the blood, and increases the breakdown of fibrin (which helps prevent blood clots).

As long as you eat a pretty healthy diet (with ample fruits and vegetables, along with whole grains), you will get a rather good supply of all of these antioxidants, except one: vitamin E. One study demonstrated that when postmenopausal women ate foods rich in vitamin E, they significantly reduced their risk for heart disease. You'll find vitamin E naturally in dark green leafy vegetables, avocados, canola oil, some nuts, whole grain cereals, and egg yolks. But the ideal amounts being shown to help manage menopausal symptoms, improve immune function, and reduce the risk of heart disease are more in the 400 IU supplement range. Therefore, by taking a supplement in addition to eating these sources of vitamin E you will make certain to have enough.

If we're going to talk about antioxidants and heart disease we've got to mention our other friend, the phytochemical (protective substances found in plant foods). One of the phytoestrogens, isoflavone (found in soy and other plant foods), for example, helps lower LDL (bad) cholesterol, and new evidence suggests it may help LDLs resist oxidation. But you can't take this in a pill—it only seems to work in food form. Scientists suspect there is some necessary component in soy protein that allows the phytochemicals to do their job properly. You can also get a supply by eating garlic, squash, apples, berries, broccoli, cabbage, carrots, citrus fruits, cucumbers, eggplant, grapes, lettuce, peppers, tomatoes, and yams.

Another powerful food weapon you have in your arsenal are the omega-3 fatty acids. They are probably best known for lowering plasma triglyceride levels in the blood. Eating three-ounce servings of fish several times a week would provide the amounts recommended by many researchers. (Your tuna sandwich counts as well.)

What about the total amount of fat? This answer could depend on your particular genetics. I think a 20- to 30-percent-calories-from-fat diet (using predominantly monounsaturated fats) is a good way to go (considering cancer and obesity prevention as well) until more is known. I personally find it difficult to lower the fat below 20 percent calories from fat, and I know most of us couldn't do this *happily* for the rest of our lives. When you eat a lower-fat diet, you are likely to automatically lower the amount of saturated fat, trans fatty acids, and omega-6s.

Q **How can I reduce the risk of osteoporosis with the foods I choose?**

There are five lifestyle risk factors for osteoporosis, three of which are diet related. The dietary risk factors are low calcium intake, high protein intake, and high caffeine intake. The other two are tobacco and alcohol use and a sedentary lifestyle.

Almost every woman knows that getting enough calcium is good for your bones. But that's only the beginning. Once you take in the calcium, you want to make sure your body holds on to as much of it as possible. To do that, you need to remember to get enough calcium-absorption enhancer foods and avoid the calcium depleter foods.

What are the calcium-absorption enhancers and what foods can I find them in?

- **Vitamin D.** Your body makes vitamin D in your skin with the help of ultraviolet light; as you age, your body makes less and less of it. You can find vitamin D in milks fortified with it, in products made with fortified milk, and in egg yolks.

- **Lactose.** All milks and some milk products such as ice cream, yogurt, and cottage cheese, contain this carbohydrate.

- **Magnesium.** Magnesium helps your bones in several ways. It increases calcium absorption from the intestines; it helps the body use vitamin D which helps your bones; and it also has a role in maintaining the completeness of bone. Magnesium is found in nuts and legumes; certain leafy green vegetables, such as broccoli and spinach; potatoes; and smaller amounts in whole-grain foods, meats, seafood, and milk.

- **Boron.** Boron helps bones by discouraging the loss of calcium through the urine. Boron is easily found in high amounts in fruits, vegetables, tubers, and legumes.

What food/drinks should I limit because they contain calcium depleters?

These are the depleters that encourage calcium loss via the kidneys and urine:

- **High protein diets.** Some researchers think that lowering the animal protein in our diet, for example, may actually reduce the amount of calcium we need.
- **Caffeine.** (Even decaffeinated coffee contains tannins that may inhibit the absorption of some minerals.)
- **Excessive sodium.**

These are the depleters that discourage calcium absorption via the intestinal tract:

- **Alcohol.** Alcohol also reduces the amount of active vitamin D formed by the body and may interfere with the bone-protecting benefits of estrogen. To top it off, alcohol may also increase calcium loss via the kidneys.
- **High phosphorus in the diet.** Excess phosphorus competes with calcium for absorption in the intestines. It's the soda and beer in the American diet that may pose a problem, if taken excessively.

There are a few other calcium depleters that I hesitate to even mention because they are found in really nutritious foods. Fiber and phytates (found in legumes, nuts and seeds, wheat bran, cellulose) can bind with some of the calcium in the intestinal tract, so it passes through unabsorbed. Whole grains, bran, and some soy products contain phytates and are high in fiber. Oxalates are organic acids that form complexes with calcium in the intestinal tract that cannot be easily absorbed. Oxalates are found in vegetables (spinach, beets, celery, eggplant, greens, okra, and squash), fruits (berries), nuts (pecans and peanuts), and also tea, coffee, and cocoa. Does this mean we should stop eating these fruits and vegetables and nuts? Or dare I say, chocolate? Absolutely not. Making sure you don't drink too much coffee or tea, though, makes a lot of sense.

Q **How much calcium do we need?**

The National Institutes of Health recommends that postmenopausal women between the ages of 50 and 64 who are not on estrogen or hormone replacement therapy, and all women over 65, consume 1,500 milligrams of calcium a day. It is recommended that postmenopausal women taking estrogen take 1,000 milligrams of calcium a day. *(If you have had calcium-containing kidney stones, you should check first with your practitioner on this, as well as receiving other calcium advice.)*

F.Y.I. **Don't get between a woman and her diet soda!**

Researchers have found a significant relationship between the amount of carbonated soda women drank and the number of bone fractures in women over 40. It isn't soda that's harmful, per se, but the huge amounts we Americans drink. Try to drink water most of the time. That is, after all, what our bodies really need. Keep sodas (even diet sodas) as a treat. I cut down to one a day when I was pregnant with my first daughter and somehow it just stuck. Have your one daily soda when you crave it the most.

Top 10 calcium-rich dairy foods

1. Yogurt, plain or flavored, low fat, 1 cup (about 350 to 415 milligrams calcium)
2. Parmesan cheese, 1 ounce shredded (350 milligrams calcium)
3. Nonfat dry milk powder, 1 ounce (350 milligrams calcium)
4. Milk, nonfat or 1-percent low fat, 1 cup (about 315 milligrams calcium)
5. Lowfat frozen yogurt, or ice milk, 1 cup (about 215-300 milligrams calcium)
6. Milk, whole or buttermilk, 1 cup (about 290 milligrams calcium)
7. Reduced fat cheeses, 1 ounce (about 200 milligrams calcium)
8. Evaporated skimmed milk, ¼ cup (185 milligrams calcium)
9. Ricotta cheese, part-skim, ¼ cup (165 milligrams calcium)
10. Cottage cheese, low fat, 1 cup (150 milligrams calcium)

Top 14 calcium-rich plant and fish foods

1. Tofu, firm, ½ cup (260 milligrams calcium)
2. Fresh soy milk (some brands), 1 cup (about 240 milligrams calcium)
3. Canned salmon, 3 ounces (about 180 to 200 milligrams calcium)
4. Collard, turnip, beet, or dandelion greens, boiled, ½ cup (80 to 180 milligrams calcium)
5. Spinach, boiled from frozen, ½ cup (about 140 milligrams calcium)
6. Blackstrap molasses, 1 tablespoon (135 milligrams calcium)

7. Ocean perch fish, 2 ounces baked or broiled (about 120 milligrams calcium)

8. Fresh spinach leaves, 2 cups chopped (about 110 milligrams calcium)

9. Broccoli, cooked from frozen, 1 cup (about 95 milligrams calcium)

10. Kale, boiled from frozen, ½ cup (90 milligrams calcium)

11. Clams, 3 ounces steamed/boiled/canned (about 80 milligrams calcium)

12. Instant oatmeal, cream of wheat, or Maypo, 1 packet (about 80 milligrams calcium)

13. Freshwater bass or rainbow trout, 3 ounces baked/broiled (75 milligrams calcium)

14. Beans—small white, navy, great northern, kidney, cooked—½ cup (60 to 80 milligrams calcium)

Q **I don't get enough calcium in my diet. What do I need to know about calcium supplements?**

This issue hits close to home. I don't like the taste of milk so I've never been an avid milk drinker. In fact, I got through pregnancy by chasing every glass of heavily iced milk down with a squirt of chocolate syrup. But I do enjoy reduced fat cheeses and lowfat yogurts on an almost daily basis. That's where I get most of my calcium.

Do try and get as much of the daily recommended calcium as you can through food. In the case of dairy products, for example, the calcium automatically comes to you in the presence of calcium-absorption enhancers such as lactose (carbohydrate in milk and some milk products) magnesium (milk contains a modest amount) and vitamin D (milks are fortified with D). Then, if need be, fill in the gap with supplements. Follow these three steps to get a good idea of how much calcium you might need to supplement.

- **Step #1:** Use the information mentioned above to guesstimate how much calcium you get from food on an average day. *(For example, I get about 800 milligrams a day.)*

- **Step #2:** Take a look at your multivitamin/mineral pill (if you take one) and add that amount of calcium to your food total. *(My supplement contains 162 milligrams per pill.)*

- **Step #3:** Subtract the amount you take in through food and your multivitamin from the amount recommended: (1,500 milligrams/day for postmenopausal women between 50 and 64 who are not on estrogen or hormone replacement therapy, and all women over 65, 1,000 milligrams/day; 1,000 milligrams/day for women age 25 to 49 (premenopausal). *(I subtracted 962 from 1,500, leaving a gap of about 500 missing milligrams.)*

Calcium rules to supplement by

- Take your calcium supplement with a meal or snack and with lots of water (to discourage constipation). When you eat a meal or snack, your body automatically releases stomach acid to start digestion. It just so happens that stomach acid is another calcium-absorption enhancer.

- Calcium is absorbed best in 250-milligram doses throughout the day. So if you are taking a multivitamin/mineral (containing around 200 milligrams of calcium), you might want to take it in the morning and then take your calcium supplement with dinner (or visa versa).

- Simply chewing calcium tablets increases calcium absorption.

- Avoid calcium supplements from "natural" sources such as bonemeal, oyster shell, or dolomite—they might contain toxic minerals such as lead or other toxic metals.

- Many people opt for calcium carbonate supplements. However calcium carbonate requires acidity to be absorbed, and it can cause gastric acid rebound (when taken on an empty stomach). So it is best to take it with meals. There are also some known side effects to calcium carbonate: kidney stones, constipation, and gas.

- Products made with calcium citrate or calcium citrate-malate are more expensive but are easier on the stomach, and the body absorbs the calcium better. Calcium citrate is also better for the elderly or anyone who is at higher risk of kidney stones. Calcium lactate or calcium gluconate are also acceptable options.

- Each different type of calcium supplement supplies a different percentage of "elemental calcium" (the actual amount of absorbable calcium), so check the label. This is the amount that you add to your daily calcium count.

- Don't take too much calcium—it can interfere with the absorption of other minerals, cause constipation, and increase your risk of urinary stone formation. Calcium supplements can also interfere with the absorption of certain medications (tetracycline for one). And besides, it's a waste of money. Studies have shown that calcium supplements weren't helpful for women who already meet their requirement for calcium.

- If you are in perimenopause and are losing a lot of blood due to frequent or heavy periods, take your multivitamin with iron at a different time than your extra calcium supplement because calcium supplements can inhibit iron absorption.

 My friends spend hundred of dollars on all sorts of special vitamins and supplements. Which ones should I consider?

Food is still the best way to get nutrients. Nature made it complete and balanced. Rarely can you take in too much of a vitamin, mineral, or phytochemical by eating whole foods. But in this busy day and age, many of us don't quite meet the recommendations for certain vitamins and minerals. Menopause is certainly no exception.

You can cover a lot of nutritional ground just by taking a really good multivitamin with minerals. It doesn't sound as glamorous as the other stuff your friends are buying, but it isn't as expensive either. And it works. For perimenopausal women, for example, it contains the 15 milligrams of zinc that may help "vitalize" vaginal tissues; it contains 100 percent Daily Value (or Recommended Daily Allowance) for the B vitamins, including B6; and it contains 400 micrograms (100 percent Daily Value) of folic acid. You'll also get some calcium and magnesium and 400 IU (100 percent Daily Value) of vitamin D to help your bones. Many multivitamins also have two other antioxidants: vitamin A (my supplement contains 40 percent as beta carotene) and some selenium.

Nearly half of the women in America take some type of vitamin-mineral supplement. A complete supplement should contain all of the B vitamins plus folic acid, for example, and all the essential vitamins and minerals. And even though we don't yet have a daily recommended amount for the mineral chromium, it is important that your supplement have at least the minimum suggested by the Recommended Daily Allowance committee—50 micrograms—because it is one of the minerals we seem to need more of as we age. It is involved in carbohydrate and fat metabolism and helps maintain blood sugar levels and possibly participates in insulin's action in the body.

The multivitamin needs not only to have the right substances, but the right amounts. You want your multivitamin with minerals to contain 100 percent of the Daily Value for most of the vitamins and minerals. You will find a few exceptions. Biotin will only be at 10 percent Daily Value because it is very expensive. Calcium or magnesium won't generally be found in amounts much greater than 25 percent Daily Value. Because they add so much bulk, our vitamins would start to resemble horse pills at the 100-percent level.

 I've heard that soy, because it is rich in phytoestrogens, may increase the risk of breast cancer if eaten in large quantities *after* menopause. What should I do?

There are lots of reasons why women (and their families for that matter) might want to eat more soy. Soy is a complete protein, and contains B vitamins, calcium, omega-3 fatty acids, isoflavone (phytoestrogens), and some fiber.

As of late, there is increasing evidence that eating soy products can help protect against some cancers, heart disease, and possibly even some of the symptoms of menopause. This protection appears to be due, at least in part, to the isoflavones (phytoestrogens) that are found in soybeans.

Plant estrogens, when eaten in foods, do seem to be protective against some cancers *before* menopause. And soy foods do seem to help many women manage some of their uncomfortable symptoms *during* menopause. But whether soy remains protective against some cancers *after* menopause is the big question. Some scientists suspect a daily diet of soy may actually slightly increase the risk of certain cancers when a woman is postmenopausal. So what should we do?

Let's not forget that soy is a whole lot more than a possible anticarcinogen. We should be eating more servings of soy just for its lipid lowering merits (heart disease is, in fact, the number one killer in America). Servings of soy appear to lower LDL cholesterol while leaving HDL (good cholesterol) alone. Some researchers speculate that eating about *25 grams (one serving) of soy protein a day could reduce one's heart disease risk by 20 percent.*

And the heart disease benefits just won't stop there. A Japanese research team found that when rabbits are fed soy milk, their LDL cholesterol oxidation is dramatically suppressed (we want to suppress LDL oxidation because it enables the cells that line the arteries to take up cholesterol, leading to plaque formation). This preliminary data only serves to give soy more stripes and health honors because preventing LDL oxidation may be as important for lowering heart disease risk as lowering cholesterol levels.

If, however, you have or have had an estrogen-sensitive tumor, and if you are postmenopausal, it is probably wise to eat soy occasionally, rather than frequently, until more is known.

For all you perimenopausal women out there though, you can get more soy in your diet by following the Tofu Tips in Chapter 4.

Q Are there certain fats that are better for you than others?

Maybe you are part of the 24 percent of the American population that is successfully eating a healthy diet. Or maybe you are part of the 23 percent that has been intending to or trying to eat a healthy diet (JADA Oct. 1998). Either way I'm sure you've come face to face with big daily decisions about...*fats*. Which cooking oil should I buy? Which margarine is best? Should I still buy butter? What if I don't want to use olive oil in my cakes and muffins?

Some of us are a little more motivated to find answers to these questions than others. A little less than a tenth of us are *very* motivated—this is the portion of U.S. adults "living" with heart disease (7.5 percent of adults in the United States have survived a heart attack or experience chest pain caused by heart disease). These same people may have ridden the fats-and-oils roller coaster of information over the years: saturated fat is bad—eat margarine; trans fatty acids are bad, too—don't eat margarine; polyunsaturated fat is good—use safflower oil; polyunsaturated fat isn't so good—switch to olive oil.

Years ago, we read that everyone should eat a lowfat diet. Lately, however, study results are proving that a very lowfat diet isn't necessarily healthful for everyone—especially one that has replaced fat with oodles of sugar (thanks to popular fat-free products that make up the difference in taste with sugar).

More and more, the research in heart disease and cancer prevention is pointing us to the new question: "What protective factors in foods and fats do I need to *add* to my diet?" Believe it or not, there do seem to be health benefits to certain fats, making them perhaps "best fats." The bottom line is, Americans want their food to taste good. In a recent study, taste was still the most important consideration in American food choices, followed by cost, nutrition, convenience, and weight control (JADA Oct. 1998). And at least some fat is needed in many dishes, some of them our favorites, to make them taste good. So because we are still going to use some fat, what fat do we use?

In the past few years, a lot of studies have helped shed some light on this whole "right fats/wrong fats" dilemma, although many questions still remain. But if you put together what we know so far, a pattern starts to emerge.

Where Americans are now

- A recent study suggests that the average American takes in an average of 5.3 grams of trans fatty acids per day, which is 2.6 percent of his or her total calories (7.4 percent of the total fat intake). This amount is likely to be higher in reality because people tend to underreport their food intakes by 20 to 40 percent (JADA Feb. 1999).
- Americans are taking in plenty of saturated fat, contributing 12.5 percent of our total calories.
- Americans eat a 1 to 6 or 1 to 10 ratio of protective omega-3 fatty acids to the more damaging omega-6s.
- Americans eat, on average, a little more than 30 percent of calories from fat.

Where Americans need to go

Some researchers suggest that Americans need to eat a 1:1 ratio of omega-3 fatty acids to omega-6s, just to even the odds for the omega-3s. To do this we need to get more omega-3s in food while drastically lowering our omega-6s. The quickest way to do this is to switch our cooking oils to canola and olive oil (away from an omega-6 vegetable oil), switch to a tub margarine with liquid canola or olive oil listed as the first ingredient (away from margarine that contains trans fatty acids), and eat omega-3-rich fish a couple times a week when possible.

The Lion Diet Heart Study, a diet study in France, tested this. One of the main things the participants did was switch to a canola oil margarine. The study found that there was a significant decrease in heart attacks and related deaths.

 ## Best Fats (and the benefits)

Omega-3

Omega-3 fatty acids help wage war against both heart disease and cancer. Omega-3s have been linked to lowering both blood pressure and serum triglyceride levels (high serum triglycerides have recently been found to be an independent risk factor for heart disease), preventing blood clots (decreasing the chance of stroke), and preventing the closing of blood vessels following vascular surgery. Omega-3s may even help increase levels of HDL (good) cholesterol. In one study eating fish two times a month decreased risk of cardiac arrest by 30 percent (compared to those who ate no fish), while eating fish even more often—once a week—decreased the risk of cardiac arrest by 50 percent.

Omega-3s have also been shown to slow or prevent cancerous tumor growth (it looks most helpful for colon and breast cancer) and reduce symptoms of inflammatory disease, as is the case with rheumatoid arthritis.

Best food sources: higher fat fishes (sardines, salmon, mackerel, anchovies, herring) along with other seafood sources (striped bass, bluefish, shark, tuna and canned tuna, rainbow trout, and pacific oysters), and some plant foods (the body converts some of the alpha-linolenic acid to one of the omega-3 fatty acids) such as flaxseed, walnuts, rapeseed (used to make canola oil), soybeans, spinach, and mustard greens.

Omega-9 fatty acids

Oleic acid is being called the "omega-9 fatty acid," and it looks like this fatty acid may reduce the development of breast cancer tumors (mammary carcinomas). Of course, we need to discover more about oleic acid, but in the meantime, you can find it in monounsaturated fat sources many of us have switched to anyway: canola and olive oil.

Monounsaturated fat

Replacing saturated fats with mostly monounsaturated fats helps minimize the unwanted decrease in the HDL (good) cholesterol that often occurs when you lower the total amount of fat in your diet. Some scientists think it is possible that monounsaturated fats also slightly reduce the risk of breast cancer. Olive oil is also rich in polyphenol antioxidants (helpful toward heart disease and cancer protection) and is possibly the only significant food source of squalenes (a substance that, in animal studies, slowed growth of colon, lung, and skin cancers). Recent studies in Greece and Spain found that women who consumed the most olive oil had a much lower risk (25- to 40-percent decrease in risk) of developing breast cancer than those who ate the least.

Best food sources: olive oil and canola oil are highest in monounsaturated fat; peanut oil has slightly less than canola oil. Although soybean oil contains more than 20 percent monounsaturated fat, 60 percent of it is poly-unsaturated fat.

Note: Polyunsaturated fat is not listed as one of the best fats because research has been associating higher levels with an increased risk of breast and ovarian cancers. And many of the vegetable oils that are rich in polyunsaturated fat are also very high in omega-6 fatty acids.

 Worst Fats (and the dangers)

Trans fatty acids

When vegetable oils are "partially hydrogenated" (which is a common process manufacturers use to make oils more solid and more stable), some of the fatty acids convert to a "trans" molecular configuration. These trans fats are particularly dangerous because they raise our LDL (bad) cholesterol blood levels while lowering our precious HDL (good) cholesterol levels. Some scientists estimate that trans fatty acids are actually two times more dangerous to our heart health than saturated fat.

Saturated fat

High amounts of saturated fat tend to raise LDL cholesterol levels in the blood and are associated with heart disease (saturated fat does not seem to reduce the HDL cholesterol levels like trans fatty acids do). Recent evidence links together diets high in saturated fat to an increased risk of several types of cancer: ovarian, colon, and breast cancer. Some association has also been shown between animal fat (a major source of saturated fat) and prostate and colon cancer in men.

Polyunsaturated fat

New animal data indicates that diets high in linoleic acid (the predominant polyunsaturated fat in the American diet) increases the risk of various cancers. Tumors grew faster in animals eating the study diet that contained more linoleic acid. The linoleic also enhanced metastasis (the spreading of cancer cells). For obvious reasons, it would be unethical to test a high polyunsaturated or linoleic acid diet on women at risk for breast cancer. But a four-year study in Sweden (including data on 61,000 women) found that women who ate the most polyunsaturated fat were 20 percent more likely to develop breast cancer than those who ate the least.

Linoleic acid not only increases the risk of human cancer, but also compromises our lipid levels. Although linoleic acid does appear to lower LDL and total cholesterol levels, linoleic acid also decreases HDL cholesterol levels. Additionally, high intakes of linoleic have been shown to increase the susceptibility of LDL cholesterol to oxidation—the primary cause of atherosclerotic plaguing.

Omega-6 fatty acids

Omega-6 fatty acids compete with the valuable omega-3s for control of many biochemical reactions in the body. When omega-6s are in a much higher proportion than omega-3s, an overproduction of hormone-like substances (prostaglandins and leukotrienes) result, encouraging plaque buildup on artery walls, disrupting the immune system, and forming blood clots.

It isn't that omega-6 fatty acids are damaging by themselves per se; it is the ratio of omega-3 to omega-6 fatty acids that has become unhealthy in the American diet.

Omega-6 fatty acids are found in corn, safflower, and sunflower oil and in foods that are manufactured with these oils.

For supermarket tips to avoid these dangerous fats, see Chapter 7.

 *Chapter 4*

The 10 Food Steps to Freedom

*T*he 10 Food Steps to Freedom are the 10 things you can start doing right now to help encourage a more comfortable perimenopause, a healthy heart, and strong bones.

These are the three main issues that many women face at this point in their lives, and that is the reason I focused on them here. These 10 steps incorporate most of the food advice you've been reading in the past three chapters. You've heard about thymptoms relief (for some women), so there is a food step reserved just for soy. You've also heard about how most beans are rich sources of phytoestrogens (and other important nutrients we need more of as we age), so there is a food step to eat more beans.

We've covered a lot of ground in Chapters 1 through 3, and this is the chapter that puts all the puzzle pieces together. You can start to see a picture forming—of a healthier way to eat and live. Many of the following food steps accomplish several important health moves at once. They aren't just beneficial for perimenopause symptom relief. Many also help the heart and bones, your mind, and your energy level. Best of all, most of the 10 food steps also help protect the body against cancer, something we are all concerned about—at any age. I have provided some of my favorite recipes in Chapter 5. Chapter 6 will help you navigate the supermarket. And Chapter 7 provides you with helpful restaurant tips. So let's get started!

Food Step #1: Eat more tofu and soy

By now we know that we should be substituting high protein plant foods, like tofu, for our high protein animal foods, at least some of the time. We also know that eating more tofu and soy products has helped some perimenopausal women. And we know that tofu and soy may help protect our heart and arteries by making the fats in our blood less damaging and plaque less likely to form. So, with this kind of winning nutritional endorsement, are we eating more tofu and soy? Heck no!

Many of us have never tasted tofu or soy, and if you aren't used to it, let's face it, it looks really strange. It is completely different from the favorite American foods, that's true. But once you have it a few times, it can be a food you enjoy, and actually crave. Take it from me. When I started this book, I had tofu on the occasion that I went to a Chinese restaurant or ate at a vegetarian friend's house. But that was about it. Today, I stand before you, a conformed tofu-ite. I won't go so far as to make cheesecake with it, but I have come to love many of the tofu and soy milk recipes you will find in Chapter 5.

Here are some easy ways to eat more tofu whether you are at home or dining out.

Turning the terror of tofu into the joy of soy

- Choose tofu dishes or substitute tofu for meat in your favorite dishes at your local Chinese restaurant.

- Enjoy miso soup at your favorite Japanese restaurant (and take a serving of miso soup home for a quick snack the next day).

- On harried mornings, make the breakfast smoothie in Chapter 6 (it uses silken tofu) and pump your fast-paced morning up with a glass full of high-powered nutrients. Although it is a breakfast drink, you won't be hungry for several hours.

- Buy baked tofu in your supermarket, and experiment with it at home (add it to salads, eat it plain, or with crackers).

- Drink chocolate, flavored, or plain soy milk. I tasted quite a few brands available to me in California and the best tasting soy milk, by far, is a *fresh* soy milk made by WhiteWave in Boulder, Colorado. It is called "Silk" Dairyless Soy Beverage and it comes in chocolate or plain in refrigerated cartons. You can find it in many health or natural food stores and you can surf WhiteWave's Web site at www.whitewave.com.

- Munch on a handful of roasted soybeans. You can buy them at a health food store or roast them yourself at home.

- Buy canned soybeans and add them to soups, chili, and casseroles.

Practical tofu tips

Tofu tends to turn really quickly. To prevent any tofu mishaps, follow the practical tips that follow:

- Check the expiration date on the package before you buy it.
- Open the package only when you are absolutely sure you are going to use it.
- Cover any unused tofu with water, cover the container with plastic wrap, then refrigerate it. Change the water almost every day until you use it up. (I suggest using it within a couple of days.)
- You can also freeze tofu. But beware that when you thaw it out, it will crumble into pieces. This is a quality you might want if you are using tofu in certain recipes, such as chili.

Food Step #2: Eat more fruits and vegetables

There are so many benefits to eating more fruits and vegetables, especially those rich in phytoestrogens and boron. Health benefits include: fiber, vitamins and minerals, antioxidants, phytochemicals, and most are naturally low in fat, sugar, and sodium.

There may be many health reasons to eat more fruits and vegetables, but there are also many *perimenopausal* reasons to eat more. Let's focus on these for a minute.

Phytoestrogens

Phyto*chemicals* are special plant chemicals that help protect our bodies' health and well-being. The phyto*estrogens* are a particular group in the general phytochemical family. Phytoestrogens are plant chemicals that are very similar in structure to estrogen and act like weak estrogens in our bodies. These weak estrogens either block or enhance estrogen action in our bodies. This all depends on whether you are currently pre-, peri-, or postmenopausal.

If your estrogen levels are high in your body *(before perimenopause),* these weak plant estrogens are thought to attach to the estrogen receptors in your body, thereby inactivating some of the more potent estrogens circulating in your body (which can possibly help decrease the development or growth of various estrogen-dependent cancers.)

If your estrogen levels are changing or decreasing *(perimenopause),* the plant estrogens act like a weaker version of estrogen—tricking your body into thinking it has more estrogen than it really does—potentially diminishing some of the discomforts caused by lower estrogen levels.

If your estrogen levels are almost nonexistent *(menopause and beyond),* then it is possible that plant estrogens increase the amount of circulating weak estrogens in the body, helping to decrease the risk of the chronic diseases (heart disease and osteoporosis) women get when they are past 60.

The one question about phytoestrogens that is still unanswered is whether higher amounts of weak plant estrogens in the body increase the growth or risk of estrogen-sensitive cancers. Until more is known, if you have or have recently had estrogen-dependent cancer, it is probably best that you *not* consume phytoestrogen-rich foods on a daily or frequent basis.

Boron

Boron is a mineral that is easy to find in some of our favorite fruits and vegetables. It also seems to increase the body's ability to hold onto estrogen. Studies done by the USDA's Human Nutrition Laboratory showed that 3 milligrams of boron from food doubled the level of circulating estrogen in *post*menopausal women.

Boron also helps keep our bones strong by decreasing the amount of calcium excreted (lost) by the body by 40 percent. In the table that follows, I've listed the boron-rich foods that also contain phytoestrogens (either isoflavones or lignans,) so they are extra helpful during perimenopause.

F.Y.I. *For your information...*

The **fruits** that do not contain phytoestrogens but are still rich in boron include: quinces, peaches, figs, sour cherries, red currants, apricots, black currants, American persimmons, bananas, mangos, cantaloupes, papayas, gooseberries, mandarin oranges, avocados, and blueberries.

The **vegetables and legumes** that do not contain phytoestrogens but are still rich in boron are: dandelions (leaf), celery roots, radishes, Brussels sprouts (leaf and stem), cowpeas, rutabagas (leaf, stem, and root), alfalfa, black beans (fruit and seed), spinach, butter beans, endive, Chinese cabbage, chicory (root), cauliflower (stem), and corn.

Make eating fruits and vegetables a habit

I think we would all eat more fruits and vegetables if we just had our mother taking care of us. We need someone to remember to buy the fruits and vegetables, someone to take the time to turn them into beautiful fruit salads or green salads, snack trays, and garnishes or tasty side dishes.

Make a point of treating yourself to more fruits and vegetables every day. Here are some ways to make fruits and vegetables a little more convenient.

- Pack your desk or car with your favorite dried fruits; they will keep for weeks.

F.Y.I. Top food sources of boron that also contain phytoestrogens

Fruits:	Vegetables and others:
plums,	cabbage (i)
prunes when dried (L)	asparagus (L)
strawberries (i)	lettuce (i)
apples (i)	iceberg lettuce (L)
tomatoes (i)	beets (L)
pears (L)	cauliflower (L)
grapes (i)	cucumbers (i)
grapefruit (i)	onions (L)
oranges (i)	carrots (i, L)
red raspberries (I)	broccoli stems (i, L)
	turnips (L)
	sweet potatoes (L)
	bell peppers (i, L)
	soybeans (i, L)
	wheat (L)

(i) = isoflavones   (L) = Lignans

- Buy baby carrots and celery sticks and put them out before dinner with a quick dip (mix some light or fat free sour cream with Ranch dressing mix or Onion dip mix).

- Take time Sunday or at the beginning or end of the work week to make a large spinach salad or vegetable-fortified lettuce salad, and store it (without dressing) in an airtight container. You can have crisp, wonderful salad as a snack or with your lunch or dinner for the next few days.

- Every few days make a point of going to your supermarket and picking out the best tasting and freshest in-season fruits. Remember to put it out as a snack for the family. Add a few slices or wedges of fruit to each lunch or dinner plate.

- With a few chops of a knife, you can turn a few pieces of fruit into a beautiful fruit salad. Drizzle lemon, pineapple, or orange juice over the top and toss to coat (the vitamin C helps prevent browning).

- Buy your favorite fruits in the winter—just buy them frozen or canned in juice or light syrup.

- Stock your refrigerator at work and home with your favorite fruit juices (make sure they are 100-percent juice). You can often buy them in individual servings so you can grab them as you are running out the door.

- Make a point to include a vegetable with your lunch.

- Make sure and enjoy vegetables when you eat out at a restaurant or deli.

Food Step #3: Eat beans more often

Eating beans more often comes quite naturally to other cultures and countries across the globe, but not in America. Often the only time many Americans eat beans is when they are eating out at a Mexican restaurant. But to give us some credit, there are a couple of traditionally American dishes that feature beans: chili and baked beans. And the farther south you go in the United States, the more likely you are to see beans on a menu, too.

Beans are a nutritionally efficient food because they have so many health benefits in one little package. They:

- appear to slow the absorption of glucose in the bloodstream, thus curbing your appetite longer. They may also cause your body to need less insulin, a major benefit for diabetics.

- are packed full of fiber.

- can contain phytoestrogens (soybeans contain isoflavones, while lentils, soybeans, kidney beans, navy beans, pinto and fava beans are rich in lignins, another kind of phytoestrogen).

- contain other beneficial phytochemicals that help protect the body from disease, including protease inhibitors, phytosterols, and saponins.

- are a lowfat source of plant protein.

- are great sources of many vitamins and minerals we need more of as we age, such as folic acid and vitamin B-6.

- are pretty good calcium sources. The following beans have about 125 milligrams calcium per 1 cup, cooked:

  - small white beans.
  - navy beans.
  - great northern beans.
  - red kidney beans.

Finally, a diet rich in bean fiber tends to significantly decrease total blood cholesterol and produce a better HDL (good) cholesterol to LDL (bad) cholesterol ratio.

Breaking down the barriers to beans

Beans give you gas. There, I said it. But there are ways around this. Add beans slowly to your diet. Eat about half a cup per day about two times a week to start. Use canned beans and rinse them well before adding them to your recipes. And try over-the-counter gas fighting remedies, such as Beano, if you continue to have a problem. Beano, for example, contains enzymes that break down the gas-producing sugars in beans.

Dry beans take too much time to soak, rinse, boil, and drain. So use canned. How hard can it be to open a can, dump the beans in a colander, and rinse? Some brands even offer lower sodium canned beans.

I don't know what to do with beans. Besides their obvious uses—adding beans to your burrito, nachos, or quesidillas, and sprinkling kidney beans in your green salad, here are few other ways to eat more beans:

- Add beans to soups, stews, or chili that you normally make at home.
- Order bean soups in restaurants.

- Buy the better-tasting canned bean soups or vegetarian chili to have around at home for a quick side dish or snack.

- Make a quick three-bean salad by just tossing a light salad dressing with three different types of canned beans. (See the recipe printed in Chapter 6.)

- Sprinkle some beans on a green salad, pasta salad, Southwestern chicken salad, or taco salad.

- Make a delicious bean dip for parties. When the party is over, keep it in the refrigerator for a quick snack.

Food Step #4: Eat more of the right fats

Yes, it is rather important to avoid eating a high-fat diet. High-fat foods are usually very high in calories and low in important nutrients, exactly the opposite of what a woman in or past perimenopause needs. But what may matter even more is whether a woman is getting too much of the wrong fats and not enough of the right fats.

To condense what we learned earlier, considering heart disease and cancer prevention, the right fats seem to be the omega-3 and the omega-9 fatty acids, which can be found mostly in monounsaturated fats (canola oil and olive oil) and fatty fish. The wrong fats seem to be the saturated fats, trans fatty acids, and too much of the omega-6 fatty acids (found in popular polyunsaturated oils).

What this means in food terms is that we need to:

- Switch to olive oil and canola oil (instead of other vegetable oils) when possible.
- Eat more fish.
- Eat less animal fat by choosing leaner meats and lower-fat dairy products and eat more plant protein (from soy, beans, and vegetables) instead of animal protein.
- Limit your intake of foods that contain high amounts of hydrogenated and partially hydrogenated oils.
- Buy "packaged" products less often, especially those high in fat, because most of them still use hydrogenated omega-6 oils.
- Avoid stick margarine. There are some better tasting tub margarines that list liquid canola oil or olive oil as the first ingredient. If you use butter, fine. Just use less and use canola oil or olive oil in cooking instead when you can.

Cooking with the right fats

If a recipe calls for vegetable oil, use canola oil. If it calls for vegetable oil and you think the flavor in olive oil would compliment the dish, and the oil wouldn't be heated to a high temperature (olive oil starts smoking and breaking down at higher temperatures), then you can even use olive oil instead. But what about the recipes that call for shortening, stick butter, or margarine? This gets a little tricky.

If you are using a lower-fat recipe from the start, that helps, because whatever fat you are using is at least being added in smaller amounts. (Check out a few of my cookbooks, *The Recipe Doctor Cookbook, Lighten Up!,* or *Chez Moi,* for some great reduced-fat recipes.)

I still occasionally use butter because that truly is the best fat to use for that particular recipe. However, I will cut it down as far as I can (substituting other high flavor/high moisture ingredients for additional fats). But if butter isn't that essential to the recipe and your original recipe calls for beating the butter, margarine, or shortening in a mixer, usually with sugar then eggs, you can switch to a margarine with liquid canola oil as the primary ingredient. Sometimes you can get away with beating part canola oil and part fat-free cream cheese or sour cream in place of the original fat. If you are just sautéing something in a pan, you can very easily switch to canola or olive oil and you can probably use less than in the original recipe, especially if you are using non-stick pans. Or you can use canola oil or olive oil cooking sprays.

Start collecting recipes (that you and your family like) that call for olive or canola oil. I made up a reduced-fat pie crust recipe that uses canola oil. I now use salad dressings that contain canola or olive oil for my vinaigrette-dependent recipes (such as green salad and pasta salad). These are the kinds of changes you can start making right now.

Food Step #5: Choose your beverages wisely

- Drink lots of water, a glass or two of milk, and a glass of orange (or other citrus), carrot, or purple grape juice every day.
- Limit coffee and caffeinated beverages, soda, and alcohol.

What you choose to quench your thirst with throughout the day can either rob your body of important nutrients or it can add them. We all know we *should* be drinking eight glasses of water a day, but few of us do. All this water keeps your urine diluted and your kidneys well flushed. As we grow older, our sense of thirst has a tendency to lessen, so we can't necessarily trust our thirst to tell us when it's time to drink water.

The other end to keeping our kidneys in the pink, so to speak, is limiting drinks that are diuretics. Caffeine and alcohol are both diuretics, which means they force our kidneys to get rid of more water than they should— encouraging dehydration. Caffeine, alcohol, and soft drinks (carbonated beverages) also don't do your bones any favors. Some lower the amount of calcium your body takes in from food and others increase the amount of calcium your body loses through the kidneys and urine.

Now, let's talk about nutrients that we can get from drinking certain beverages. Having a glass of juice a day is an easy habit for most of us to get into. So pick your juice wisely.

Orange juice, grapefruit juice, and other citrus fruits

Citrus fruits, in general, contain more than a hundred phytochemicals (terpenes and carotenoids, just to name two). Grapefruit and orange juice contain the phytochemical limonoids that can act to inhibit tumor formation. Pink grapefruit contains lycopene, which has been shown to reduce tumor activity. One orange is thought to contain around 170 different phytochemicals. What happens to these when an orange is "juiced"? Many of them remain, especially if you buy juice with pulp.

Orange juice. There are some calcium-fortified orange juices and orange juice blends out there that can really come in handy when you don't like to drink (or can't drink) milk. Calcium-fortified orange or orange-tangerine juice gives us a nice dose of calcium along with our vitamin C and folic acid. (For information on milk and other calcium-rich foods, see Food Step #7.)

Carrot juice. It takes some getting used to, but carrot juice can be very refreshing, not to mention very nutritious. For example, carrots contribute at least three important phytochemicals (phenolic acids, terpenes, carotenoids—including beta carotene.)

Purple grape juice. Okay, I never thought I would be writing a book where I was telling people to drink grape juice. But the truth is there are some powerful phytochemicals to be found in these purple gems. In fact, the same beneficial antioxidants that are in red wine are also found in nonalcoholic grape juice. Grapes also contain phenolic acids (which are a class of phytochemicals).

Food Step #6: Be a grazer not a gorger

In America we have this whole meal thing backwards. We burn most of our fuel during daylight hours but eat most of our calories in the evening. Our most popular time to snack is the worst possible time to snack, metabolically speaking.

Many women eat their largest meal of the day at the end of the day—dinner. And many women eat light during the time our body needs fuel the most—breakfast and lunch. When you do this, your body is more likely to store much of those calories as body fat because your body is metabolizing all those dinner calories at a time when you are burning the fewest calories.

You see, the food calories in your meal or snack turn into energy that circulates in your blood stream about 30 to 60 minutes later, peaking around one and a half to two hours after eating. What is happening two hours after we eat dinner at 6 or 7 p.m.? Sleep? Television watching? Internet surfing? None of the those activities require a whole lot of food fuel. That's why this food step to freedom focuses on not just eating small, frequent meals, but also eating light at night.

Many of us overeat in the evening because perhaps we deprive ourselves during the day, or because we're at home, we're around the kitchen, we're watching television. It doesn't help that many of us are preparing a big family meal for dinner most of the time. But if you slowly eat dinner, just until you are comfortable, you are more likely to avoid eating extra calories. You are more likely not to overeat at dinner if you ate lunch and had an afternoon snack. Studies have proven that, for most people, the longer the gap between a previous meal or snack and dinner, the larger the dinner. That makes sense doesn't it?

Some studies have shown that people who eat small, frequent meals throughout the day tend to eat fewer total calories and fat grams at the end of the day, compared to people who eat large, infrequent meals. But here's another potential weight-loss payoff: You burn more calories digesting, absorbing, and metabolizing food when you spread it out through the day. Each time you eat, the digestion process kicks into gear. Each time it starts, it burns calories. And we're not talking small potatoes here, either. This increase in metabolism that occurs during the digestion, absorption, and metabolism of carbohydrates, fat, and protein, burns 5 to 10 percent of the total calories we eat in a day!

Following are some of the health benefits to eating small, frequent meals (grazing):

- Prevents wide swings in blood glucose (when your glucose levels drop, you feel tired).
- Keeps you from getting overly hungry.
- Minimizes extra calories that are likely to be converted to fat storage.
- Is easier on the stomach and leaves you more energetic after eating.
- Increases the amount of calories you burn digesting, absorbing, and metabolizing food.

4 steps to eating light at night

Eating big dinners is a tough habit to break, especially if your family is accustomed to it. But with some changes that you incorporate a little at a time, you can eat a light and comfortable dinner instead of a heavy full one.

- **Step 1.** Serve lower fat dinners and desserts as often as possible.
- **Step 2.** Serve small to moderate portions at dinner and dessert. Generally, if you ate small, frequent meals through the day (eating when hungry and stopping when comfortable), you can be satisfied with a moderate portion at dinner.
- **Step 3.** Select food choices for evening meals that lend themselves to lightness, such as all-in-one dishes, and hearty soups and dinner salads.
- **Step 4.** Discourage late-night snacking and big desserts. Many people eat at night because

they are bored. Instead of eating, keep your-self busy with other activities that interest you: a relaxing bath, listening to favorite music, reading a good book, catching up with phone calls to friends and family, or even ex-ercising (but make sure you don't exercise too close to bedtime).

Food Step #7: Eat calcium-rich foods every day

There are lots of ways to get your calcium: from vegetables, soy, cow's milk, fortified orange juice, even tablets. When we think of calcium, though, most of us think of milk. But what if you don't like (or can't drink) milk?

Alternative calcium sources

You can reach the 1,000 to 1,500 milligrams of cal-cium target from food, even if you don't drink milk. It's tough, but not impossible. Following are some suggestions; try the ones that appeal to you.

- Make your instant or homemade oatmeal or another hot cereal with milk instead of using water.
- Order a decaf latte made with non- or lowfat milk.
- Drink a glass of lowfat milk (or soy milk) as a snack sometime during your day, add some chocolate syrup and ice cubes to make it taste better. You will get around 300 milligrams calcium along with the calcium-absorption enhancers: lactose, vitamin D, and a little magnesium.

- Take a vitamin-mineral supplement that contains 100 percent of the Daily Value for vitamin D and some calcium (around 25 percent Daily Value).
- Eat a leafy green vegetable or bean dish often (see Food Steps 2 and 3). One cup of broccoli, for example, provides 180 milligrams calcium.
- Try some great-tasting lowfat yogurt, reduced fat cheese or cottage cheese. One cup of lowfat flavored yogurt would add 345 milligrams calcium to your daily total. Dress yogurt up by sprinkling raisins, dried cranberries, or granola over the top. Stir in fresh fruit, like berries, into lemon or vanilla flavors. Make a quick yogurt parfait with light whipped topping or light whipped cream and layers of fruit, cereal, or graham cracker or cookie crumbs.
- Drinking a cup of chocolate soy milk a day won't give you the calcium-absorption enhancer lactose (milk sugar), but it will give you 30 percent of the Daily Value for calcium *and* vitamin D. See the recipe for Iced Mocha (soy milk) latte in Chapter 6.
- Enjoy cream soups (even canned) using lowfat milk instead of cream.
- Buy orange juice fortified with calcium. Some manufacturers, Minute Maid for example, make individual juice boxes in a variety of flavors (grape, cherry, apple) that are also fortified with calcium. Freeze a few of these boxes and take them along on bike or hiking trips or on car trips. A few hours later, they are still cold and refreshing.

What if you are lactose-intolerant?

Lactose is the carbohydrate (sugar) in milk. It must be broken down by the enzyme lactase in the intestinal tract before it can be absorbed into the bloodstream. However, some of use don't make enough of this enzyme to do the job properly (due to genetics, age, or gastrointestinal distress). What happens to all of this undigested milk sugar? The excess lactose stays in the intestinal tract, fermenting and drawing water into the intestinal tract, which can cause everything from gas and bloating to nausea and diarrhea.

Some people can handle a little lactose; some can't handle any. Assuming you know how much you can handle, here are some tips that may help you:

- Eat smaller servings of dairy several times a day instead of one large serving.

- Eat dairy products with a meal or in a recipe with other ingredients to dilute the concentration of lactose.

- Eat aged natural cheeses, such as cheddar and parmesan; they tend to have less lactose than other cheese because of the production and aging processes.

- Eat fermented milk products, such as yogurt because they contain active bacterial enzymes that can help you break down some of the lactose.

- Buy lactose-reduced milk to drink as a beverage or use in cooking.

- Rely on other calcium-rich foods (nondairy), such as soy milk, tofu, spinach, blackstrap molasses, greens, broccoli, and beans.

Calcium-rich foods

The following table lists calcium-rich foods and the amount of calcium per serving they contribute to your diet.

Food Source	Serving size	Total calcium
Yogurt, plain, nonfat or lowfat	1 cup	400mg
nonfat "light" flavored yogurt	1 cup	350 to 400mg
Parmesan cheese, shredded	1 ounce	350 to 400mg
nonfat dry milk powder	1 ounce	350 to 400mg
yogurt, lowfat, flavored,	1 cup	290 to 350mg
oatmeal made with lowfat milk	¾ cup	290 to 350mg
milk, nonfat, lowfat, or whole	1 cup	290 to 350mg
lowfat frozen yogurt	1 cup	290 to 350mg
buttermilk	8 ounces	200 to 290 mg
spinach, boiled	1 cup	200 to 290 mg
reduced fat cheese	1 ounce (¼ cup grated)	200 to 290 mg
tofu, firm	½ cup	200 to 290 mg
cheese pizza	1 slice	200 to 290 mg
ice milk	1 cup	200 to 290 mg
black-eyed peas, boiled	1 cup	200 to 290 mg
canned salmon	3 ounces	200 to 290 mg
macaroni and cheese	1 cup	200 to 290 mg
lowfat processed American cheese	1 slice	150 to 200 mg
evaporated skim milk	¼ cup	150 to 200 mg
pink salmon with bones, canned	3 ounces	150 to 200 mg
collard greens, boiled	½ cup	150 to 200 mg
ricotta cheese, part-skim	¼ cup	150 to 200 mg
lowfat cottage cheese	1 cup	150 to 200 mg
instant oatmeal, fortified	1 packet	150 to 200 mg

Food Source	Serving size	Total calcium
spinach, boiled	½ cup	100 to 150 mg
fresh spinach leaves	2 cups	100 to 150 mg
turnip greens, boiled	½ cup	100 to 150 mg
pudding made with milk	½ cup	100 to 150 mg
blackstrap molasses	1 tbs	100 to 150 mg
ocean perch, baked or broiled	3 ounces	100 to 150 mg
hot cocoa (check brand)	1 packet	100 to 150 mg
broccoli, cooked	1 cup	50 to 100 mg
kale, boiled	½ cup	50 to 100 mg
boy choy, boiled	½ cup	50 to 100 mg
baked beans, homemade	½ cup	50 to 100 mg
dandelion greens, cooked	½ cup	50 to 100 mg
freshwater bass, baked or broiled	3 ounces	50 to 100 mg
rainbow trout, baked or broiled	3 ounces	50 to 100 mg
cream of wheat or Maypo	½ cup	50 to 100 mg
small white beans, boiled or canned	½ cup	50 to 100 mg
navy beans, boiled or canned	½ cup	50 to 100 mg
great northern beans, boiled or canned	½ cup	50 to 100 mg
red kidney beans, boiled or canned	½ cup	50 to 100 mg
shrimp, baked or broiled	3 ounces	50 to 100 mg
pacific halibut, steamed	3 ounces	50 to 100 mg
Dinginess crab, steamed	3 ounces	50 to 100 mg

Food Step #8: Avoid high fat/high sugar foods to minimize calories

At this time in your life, preventing weight gain is really important. Now more than ever, we need to minimize any extra calories, especially those from high fat and high sugar foods.

Sugar...Ah, honey honey

Far be it for me, a confessed chocoholic, to deprive women of their daily dose of chocolate and other sweets. The point of this food step is to minimize high sugar foods. That doesn't mean you can't have any. There is a place for sweets and treats in our daily diet, just make it a small place.

I'm afraid many Americans have increased their intake of sugar in their well-intentioned efforts to reduce fat. Many of the fat-free cookies and snack foods now available have just as many calories as the regular version. Unfortunately, the fat has been replaced with sugar in various forms: high fructose, corn syrup, or honey.

Too much sugar in your daily diet can cause your blood sugar to spike, which stimulates the pancreas to release more insulin (a hormone). An excess of insulin can cause all sorts of problems. It accelerates the conversion of calories into triglycerides (fats in the blood). It stimulates a liver enzyme to make more cholesterol. It stimulates the enzyme that increases the uptake of fat from the bloodstream into fat in the body's cells. It may make your arterial walls more sticky (attracting plaque).

Where has all the sugar gone?

Soft drinks are the single biggest source of sugar, 21 percent of our refined sugar intake. We also get a large portion of our sugar from the following: 18 percent from sweets including syrups, jellies, jams, ices, popsicles, and table sugar; 13 percent from bakery desserts including cakes, cookies, pies, pastries, and sweet crackers; 10 percent of our refined sugar intake comes from milk products (ice cream, puddings, and yogurts); 6 percent comes from breads and grains. Breakfast cereals add up to 5 percent.

Food Step #9: Add flaxseed to your diet

I'll admit that I'm a little nervous about making flaxseed, a food supplement, a food step to freedom. Flaxseed is just now being studied in humans, mostly for its blood-lipid lowering benefits and tumor-reducing properties with some types of cancer. (It seems to be so effective in reducing estrogen and lowering breast cancer risk that it is now being tested clinically to shrink breast cancer tumors before surgery on women just diagnosed with the cancer.) We will know much more about flaxseed's health benefits in the coming years.

Flaxseed has actually been around and has been used by humans as both food and medicine for hundreds of years. Flaxseed was cataloged and described by physician Nicholas Culpeper in the 1600s in his book, *Complete Herbal*: "Flaxseed is of great use against inflammations, tumors and imposthumes, and is frequently put into fomentations and cataplasms" (abscesses, compresses, and poultices).

What is it about the flaxseed that might be responsible for all this? We know that flaxseed is an extraordinary source of the phytoestrogen lignans, containing 75 to 800 times as much as other plant sources, and it is also packed with the plant form of omega-3 fatty acids, alpha-linolenic acid. In fact, about half of the oil in flaxseed is alpha-linolenic acid.

Lignans are thought to lower cancer risk by blocking some effects of the estrogen your body naturally produces. They are shaped like the human version of estrogen and they may be able to grab onto breast cells, preventing your own estrogen from attaching. Lignans, though, won't stimulate cancerous breast cells to grow.

Lignans are also thought to boost production of a substance that holds onto human estrogen and carries it out of the body. And if that wasn't enough, they are also considered to act as antioxidants, protecting healthy cells from free radicals in the body.

F.Y.I. *How much flax is enough?*

Some researchers say 1 level teaspoon is enough, others recommend 1 tablespoon. Researcher Lilian Thompson, Ph.D., with the University of Toronto, says that in addition to a healthy diet, 1 to 2 tablespoons of flaxseed a day may protect us. Certainly working up to a teaspoon of flaxseed a few times a week is a moderate approach to take until more is known on the ideal daily dose. The amount currently being studied on women at high risk for breast cancer is 2 tablespoons of ground flaxseed. Each tablespoon will add about 47 calories, 2.5 grams fat and 2.7 grams fiber (one-third of which is soluble).

But you can't just start off with a tablespoon. **Some people are highly allergic to flax, so start with one-quarter teaspoon a day and increase the amount gradually if you don't have a reaction.** Another reason you want to start off slowly is that flaxseed, which is high in fiber, can cause gassiness and bloating if you aren't used to it.

The omega-3s in flaxseed help prevent blood clots that might lead to heart attacks, according to University of Toronto nutrition researcher, Stephen Cunnane, Ph.D. The omega-3s do this by helping make platelets less "sticky" or less likely to stick together, thus avoiding a chain reaction that leads to a blood clot.

Flaxseed is at the very least a good source of soluble fiber (the type of fiber that blends with water to form a gel-like mixture in the intestines), which may help lower cholesterol. When women in Cunnane's study added about 2 tablespoons of ground flax to their daily diet for four weeks, their total cholesterol fell 9 percent and their LDL (bad) cholesterol dropped 18 percent; HDL (good) cholesterol stayed the same. These same results were also found in a different study conducted by researchers in the United States.

Flaxseed, after being supplemented in a diet for just one month, may also make our arteries more flexible, something that would potentially lead to a decreased risk of heart attack and stroke.

Lilian Thompson, a nutrition scientist at the University of Toronto, has conducted research on flaxseed and animals for more than a decade. When Thompson exposed female rats to a carcinogen, after only seven weeks, the rats on the flaxseed-supplemented diet had significantly fewer and smaller mammary tumors than the group fed a standard diet. And male rats fed flaxseed were half as likely to develop colon cancer as those who ate regular rat chow.

So, in test-tube and animal studies it looks like flaxseed, probably because of its high phytoestrogen lignan content, may be helpful in shrinking existing breast and colon cancer tumors and stopping new ones from forming.

The future of flax looks very bright. Other benefits of flaxseed being suggested include the following: The oil in flaxseed, which contains antioxidants, may stimulate the immune system, and levels of vitamin D, calcium, and magnesium (all benefiting the bones) are also favorably affected. The omega-3 fatty acids found in flaxseed seems to have an anti-inflammatory effects on patients with rheumatoid arthritis (reducing morning stiffness and joint tenderness).

What do you need to know when you buy and store flaxseed? See Chapter 7 for flax-buying tips. In Chapter 6, you'll find two quick recipes for using flaxseed.

Food Step #10: Exercise, exercise, exercise

I realize exercise isn't a food, so technically it shouldn't be a "food step." But it is tied into your diet, and there are *so* many benefits of exercise during menopause that it deserves to be included in these 10 important steps. When you exercise regularly, you just plain feel better (and you look better, too). You burn more calories and you increase your muscle mass, which increases your metabolic rate. And that's just the beginning.

Exercising during menopause will help decrease blood cholesterol levels, decrease bone loss, improve your ability to deal with stress, improve circulation, improve heart function and improve oxygen and nutrient use in all body tissues.

The one health benefit almost all women will probably be most impressed with is it's weight loss and weight maintenance benefits. Menopause is one of the cases where almost everyone, thin or curvaceous, finds themselves concerned about preventing weight gain. One study showed that both thin and overweight women gained about the same number of pounds between the ages of 42 and 53. The researchers found that most women experienced considerable weight gain during their 40s. They suggest this is a result of the age-related reduction in metabolic rate and/or the drop in physical activity. Exercise is one of your best defenses. Women who have the lowest exercise levels tend to gain the most weight.

Make exercise a priority. Start making it a habit. Get a schedule going, such as walking with a neighbor on Tuesdays and Thursdays, or going to an exercise class on Mondays and Wednesdays. Get whatever help you need to make it happen. It's that important.

Exercise recommendations

If you are currently sedentary and you want to start exercising just enough to improve your chances against chronic diseases, try the following guidelines. But remember, before starting any exercise program, consult your physician.

Frequency: two to three times a week.
Intensity: 40-percent maximum heart rate.
Duration: 15 to 30 minutes.

If you want to be physically fit, try the following:

Frequency: four times a week.
Intensity: 70- to 90-percent maximum heart rate.
Duration: 15 to 30 minutes.

If you specifically want to lose weight, try the following:

Frequency: five times a week.
Intensity: 45- to 60-percent maximum heart rate.
Duration: 45 to 60 minutes.

Resistance training recommendations: Perform one set of eight to 12 repetitions of eight to 10 exercises that condition the major muscle groups at least two days a week minimum.

Follow the 10 Food Steps to Freedom and you will do your body a great service. You will slow the aging of the skeleton and the kidneys. You will eat more antioxidants, phytochemicals, phytoestrogens, and fiber. You will keep your energy constant by preventing extreme hunger and overeating. You will be less likely to eat more calories than you actually need. You will be less likely to put on extra pounds. You will increase the nutrients you need more of as you age. The bottom line is you will be doing what you can to make yourself more comfortable during perimenopause while enhancing your immune system and reducing your risk of heart disease, some types of cancer, and osteoporosis. It doesn't get much better than that.

 **Chapter 5**

The 20 Recipes You Can't Live Without

$\mathcal{I}$n this chapter, you will find some recipes that will help you take some of the hardest food steps to freedom while maintaining the joy of eating. You'll find recipes that could make tofu and soy milk daily treats.

The recipes you will find here have all been taste-tested. I handed out samples of the Tofu Chili at a nearby supermarket one evening during the dinner rush hour. People who had never tasted tofu before or had a preconceived reaction to it really loved it—even kids and teenagers. Many of the taste-testers requested some of the recipes!

What I found when I browsed through the popular tofu cookbooks was that many of the recipes were time- and ingredient-intensive. What women I spoke with said they needed most of all was quick tofu and soy milk recipes, so that's what you'll find here.

I hope that what I did for tofu and soy milk, I also did for beans, fruits, and vegetables. These are recipes that you can whip up on a near daily basis. They are, by no means, the answer to all your recipe woes, but this chapter will certainly give you a friendly nudge in the right direction.

Note: The following is a key to the abbreviations used in the recipes: tablespoon (tbs.); teaspoon (tsp.); grams (g); milligrams (mg); Daily Value (DV).

Quick and easy soy milk recipes

Soy milk, when you are accustomed to cow's milk, can take a bit of getting used to. The following soy milk recipes will taste great, but only if you use great tasting soy milk. If you've found one you like, stick with it. If you haven't, read the suggestions on buying soy milk in Chapter 6.

Note: For the soy milk recipes that follow, I used Silk soy milk by WhiteWave. The nutritional information reflects the use of this brand.

 ### Iced Mocha

- ¾ cup chocolate soy milk
- 3 to 4 tbs. chilled decaffeinated concentrated coffee, espresso, or very strong coffee
- 1 tbs. chocolate syrup (for additional chocolate flavor, if needed)
- about 6 ice cubes

Put all ingredients in food processor or blender. Pulse to crush ice and blend the ingredients into a smooth drink (makes one drink).

Per serving: 81 calories, 4 g protein, 13 g carbohydrate, 2 g fat, 0 g saturated fat, 0 mg cholesterol, 1 g fiber, 71 mg sodium. Calories from fat: 21%.

Vitamin A: 8% DV, Calcium: 23% DV, Vitamin D: 23%, Vitamin B12: 38% DV.

Mocha Soy Milk Latte

- ½ cup chocolate soy milk
- ½ cup decaffeinated double strength coffee
- a squirt of whipped cream (optional)
- cocoa or cinnamon (optional)

1. Begin brewing extra strong coffee. (Use twice as much ground coffee to brew double strength coffee.)
2. Meanwhile, add chocolate soy milk to large microwave-safe coffee mug and heat on high power in microwave until hot (about 1 to 2 minutes).
3. Add hot double strength coffee to mug with chocolate soy milk. Top with a squirt of whipped cream. Sprinkle cocoa or ground cinnamon on top, if desired (makes one latte).

Per serving: 54 calories, 2.5 g protein, 8.5 g carbohydrate, 1.2 g fat, 0 g saturated fat, 0 mg cholesterol, 0.5 g fiber, 47 mg sodium. Calories from fat: 21%.
Vitamin A: 5% DV, Calcium: 15% DV, Vitamin D: 15 % DV, Vitamin B12: 25% DV.

 ## *Instant Soy Oatmeal*

- 1 packet maple and brown sugar-flavored instant oatmeal
- $^2/_3$ cup Silk (fresh in 1-quart cartons) 1% fat Dairyless Soy Beverage

1. Empty packet into microwave-safe bowl.
2. Add soy milk and stir.
3. Microwave on high power 2 to 3 minutes.
4. Stir (makes one serving).

Per serving: 213 calories, 8 g protein, 39 g carbohydrate, 4 g fat, 0 g saturated fat, 0 mg cholesterol, 3 g fiber, 304 mg sodium. Calories from fat: 16%.
Vitamin A: 27% DV, Calcium: 30% DV, Folic Acid: 20% DV, Vitamin B12: 33% DV, Vitamin B6: 20% DV.

 ## Chocolate Soy Pudding

- 2 cups chocolate soy milk (fresh in 1-quart cartons), cold
- 1 box (about 3.9 ounces) instant chocolate pudding
- 1 envelope Knox unflavored gelatin
- 2 tbs. cold water
- 2 tbs. boiling hot water

1. Put the chocolate soy milk and instant chocolate pudding mix in mixing bowl. Beat with mixer on low speed for 2 minutes.

2. In a small bowl, add unflavored gelatin to the cold water, and let sit for 1 minute. Then stir in the boiling water and stir until mixture is relatively clear (about 1 minute).

3. Add the dissolved gelatin into the pudding mixture in mixing bowl and beat on low speed until blended. Divide into 4 serving bowls and chill about 15 minutes (makes four small servings).

Per serving: 160 calories, 4 g protein, 36.5 g carbohydrate, 2 g fat, 0 g saturated fat, 0 mg cholesterol, 0.5 g fiber, 250 mg sodium. Calories from fat: 10%.
Vitamin A: 5% DV, Calcium: 15% DV, Vitamin B12: 25% DV.

Microwave Tapoica Pudding

- ¼ cup sugar
- 3 tbs. Minute-brand Tapioca
- 2¾ cups soy milk (fresh soy milk in cartons tastes best)
- ¼ cup Egg Beaters egg substitute
- 1½ tsp. vanilla extract

1. Mix sugar, tapioca, soy milk, and egg substitute in large microwavable bowl. Cook on high power until mixture comes to a full boil (about 12 to 15 minutes), making sure to stir every few minutes.
2. Stir in vanilla extract and let cool 20 minutes; stir. Spoon into dishes and serve warm or cold. Store in refrigerator (makes four servings). For a creamier pudding, place plastic wrap over pudding while it is cooling, then stir.

Per serving: 135 calories, 6 g protein, 22 g carbohydrate, 3 g fat, 0 g saturated fat, 0 mg cholesterol, 2 g fiber, 45 mg sodium. Calories from fat: 20%.
Vitamin A: 5 RE, Vitamin E: 0 mg, Calcium: 18 mg, Folic Acid: 3 mcg.

Learning to love tofu

When it comes to eating tofu, you have two choices. You can hide it or you can flaunt it. In many Chinese dishes, such as "braised tofu and vegetables," the glorious bean curd is flaunted. Or you can, with the slight of hand, whip it up with other ingredients so it isn't totally obvious you are eating it. You'll find both types of recipes here.

Everyone has his or her own "TAI," or "Tofu Acceptance Index." Some people are more accepting of tofu, tofu products, and tofu recipes—the beanier the better. Others, and you know who you are, see a slab of tofu and run screaming in the other direction. I'm somewhere in between. I like to just call it like it is and eat it—baked, broiled, or stir-fried. I can't explain it; there is just something about the very idea of tofu cheesecake or tofu nonegg salad, for example, that makes me cringe.

But I spent days creating and testing some great-tasting tofu recipes to arm you with a soybean arsenal that I hope will keep you happy and relatively hot-flash free for a couple of years.

 ## Quick Tofu Chili

You can make a Crockpot variation of this recipe to free yourself from standing in front of the stove. Follow the sauté directions in step #1; then, in step #2, add all remaining ingredients (including the beans) to the Crockpot. Cover and cook on low for eight hours or on high for three to four hours.

- 2 tsp. canola oil
- 1 large onion, chopped
- 1 tbs. garlic, minced or chopped (or an entire bulb of roasted garlic*)
- 14 ounces firm tofu, rinsed and drained; cut into ½-inch cubes
- 1 pasilla pepper, seeded and minced (or 2 jalapeno chilies)
- 28-ounce can premium tomatoes
- ¼ cup tomato paste
- 1 green, red, or yellow bell pepper, chopped

- 2 large carrots, chopped
- 1½ tsp. ground cumin
- ¼ tsp. salt (optional)
- ¼ tsp. cayenne pepper (or to taste)
- 2 15-ounce cans pinto beans, drained
- ½ cup grated reduced fat sharp cheddar cheese

1. Heat oil in heavy, large, nonstick saucepan over medium heat. Add onion, garlic, pasilla pepper or chilies and tofu. Sauté until onions are translucent (about 6 minutes).

2. Add tomatoes with any juices, tomato paste, bell pepper, carrots, cumin, salt (if desired), and cayenne pepper. Bring to simmer, cover, and cook about 20 minutes, stirring frequently. Add the beans and cook 15 minutes longer.

3. Ladle chili into bowls and sprinkle cheese over the top (makes six cups).

Per serving: 273 calories, 17 g protein, 39.5 g carbohydrate, 7 g fat, 1.7 g saturated fat, 5 mg cholesterol, 10 g fiber, 760 mg sodium. Calories from fat: 22%.

Vitamin A: 978 RE, Vitamin C: 60 mg, Vitamin E: 1.9 mg, Calcium: 306 mg, Folic Acid: 144 mcg.

* If you happen to love roasted garlic, try this variation. To roast an entire bulb of garlic: Snip off the tops with kitchen shears, lay bulb on a sheet of foil, drizzle about ½ teaspoon of olive oil over the top, wrap up bulb in foil, and bake in 375-degree oven for about 30 minutes. Once cool, press out garlic cloves (they should be mushy) into the tofu chili along with the tomatoes and other spices.

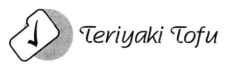 # *Teriyaki Tofu*

This recipe is addicting. If having a tofu serving a day helps you, this recipe alone could get you through menopause. Just make a batch every few days.

- 14 ounces firm tofu
- 6 tbs. light soy sauce
- 1 tsp. sesame oil
- 1 tsp. sesame seeds
- 2 tbs. sugar
- ½ cup *plus* 2 tbs. apple juice
- 1 clove garlic, crushed or minced
- 1 tsp. fresh ginger, finely minced (or ¼ tsp. ground ginger)

1. Cut the block of tofu vertically into 10 slices.
2. In small bowl, blend remaining ingredients to make teriyaki sauce. Pour sauce into a 9 x 9-inch baking pan.
3. Arrange tofu slices in sauce. Turn slices over to coat with sauce. Broil 5 to 10 minutes, then flip tofu slices over and broil 5 to 10 minutes longer (makes four servings).

Note: Serve tofu by itself, with noodles, steamed rice, or crackers.

Per serving: 135 calories, 8.5 g protein, 13 g carbohydrate, 6 g fat, 0 g saturated fat, 0 mg cholesterol, 1.5 g fiber, 770 mg sodium. Calories from fat: 37%.
Vitamin A: 9 RE, Vitamin C: 1 mg, Vitamin E: 0 mg, Calcium: 121 mg, Folic Acid: 16 mcg.

Joe's Tofu Breakfast Special

- 2 tsp. canola oil
- 6 ounces soft tofu
- 1 tsp. garlic, minced or chopped
- ½ tsp. ground sage
- pepper to taste
- $^{1}/_{3}$ cup coarsely chopped onions (optional)
- 1½ cups Ore-Ida Country Style Hash Browns, thawed
- ¾ cup thawed frozen spinach (gently squeeze excess water out)
- ¾ cup Egg Beaters egg substitute

1. Coat a large, heavy, nonstick frying pan with the canola oil.
2. Add tofu, garlic, sage, pepper, and onions and cook over medium heat until tofu and onions are just starting to brown.
3. Add hash browns (whole) and continue cooking, stirring frequently, until hash browns are lightly browned. Add spinach and egg substitute. Keep stirring until egg is cooked throughout. Serve with ketchup if desired (makes two servings).

Per serving: 252 calories, 20 g protein, 26 g carbohydrate, 9 g fat, 1 g saturated fat, 0 mg cholesterol, 4.5 g fiber, 222 mg sodium. Calories from fat: 30%.
Vitamin A: 562 RE, Vitamin C: 20 mg, Vitamin E: 2 mg, Calcium: 262 mg, Folic Acid: 102 mcg.

BBQ Tofu

I like to eat this BBQ tofu by itself, but you put it on a bun and make a sandwich, or chop it up and mix it into salad or stir-fry. Try using hickory chips when you barbecue for even more flavor.

- 9 ounces lowfat, firm nigari tofu (or other firm or extra firm tofu)
- ¼ cup of your favorite barbecue sauce **OR**
- ¼ cup of your favorite olive oil vinaigrette or Italian salad dressing

1. Cut piece of tofu in half to make two slices each about ½-inch thick.
2. Add tofu to zip-lock bag and pour in barbecue sauce or vinaigrette. Press bag to release any air and seal. Marinate in refrigerator for 30 minutes or longer.
3. Put on hot barbecue and grill about 3 inches from coals for about 2 minutes each side (makes two servings).

Per serving: 128 calories, 18 g protein, 9 g carbohydrate, 2.3 g fat, 0 g saturated fat, 0 mg cholesterol, 4.5 g fiber, about 100 mg sodium. Calories from fat: 16%.
Vitamin A: 3% DV, Calcium: 9% DV.

 # Tofu, Broccoli, and Mushroom Burrito

- 1 tsp. olive oil
- 2 tsp. garlic, minced or chopped
- 1 cup mushroom slices
- 1 cup finely chopped broccoli
- 3 ounces baked tofu (any flavor), finely cubed

- $^2/_3$ cup cooked rice or Spanish rice
- 2 tbs. fresh cilantro, chopped (optional)
- 2 green onions, finely chopped
- ½ cup shredded reduced fat Monterey Jack cheese
- 2 baby burrito flour tortillas (about 68 grams each)

1. Add olive oil to heavy nonstick medium sauce-pan or frying pan. Add garlic, mushroom slices, and broccoli and sauté over medium heat for a few minutes, or until mushrooms start to brown. Stir in tofu, cooked rice, cilantro, and green onions and continue to cook a minute or so (until tofu and rice are nice and hot).

2. Place one of the tortillas on a paper towel and sprinkle half the cheese evenly over the top. Microwave on high for about 45 seconds to soften tortilla and start to melt cheese. Spread half of the tofu mixture in center and roll up like a burrito. Repeat with remaining tortilla, cheese, and tofu mixture. (Makes two.)

Per burrito: 486 calories, 26 g protein, 64.5 g carbohydrate, 13 g fat, 4.5 g saturated fat, 15 mg cholesterol, 4.5 g fiber, 905 mg sodium. Calories from fat: 24%.
Vitamin A: 175 RE, Vitamin C: 44 mg, Vitamin E: 0.7 mg, Calcium: 327 mg, Folic Acid: 48 mcg.

 ## Tofu Cream Cheese Spread

- 3 ounces baked tofu (any flavor)
- ½ cup light cream cheese
- 2 green onions, chopped
- pepper to taste
- 2 whole grain bagels, cut in half (or any other type of bagel or bread)

1. Add tofu, cream cheese, and green onions to small food processor and pulse until creamy and well blended. Add pepper to taste.
2. Spread on bagels or fresh bread. (makes two bagel sandwiches.)

Per bagel: 297 calories, 21 g protein, 38.5 g carbohydrate, 7.5 g fat, 3.3 g saturated fat, 20 mg cholesterol, 6.5 g fiber, 780 mg sodium. Calories from fat: 22%.
Vitamin A: 280 RE, Vitamin C: 5 mg, Vitamin E: 1.5 mg, Calcium: 139 mg.

 Creamy Pesto Pasta

If you don't tell dinner guests that this recipe is made with tofu, they will never know it. All they will know is that it is the creamiest pesto sauce they have ever had. I love this dish with slices of lean turkey or chicken sausage links that have been cooked and cut into thin slices.

If you have some tofu pesto sauce left over, it makes a wonderful filling for stuffed mushroom appetizers. Spoon 1 teaspoon to 2 tablespoons of the pesto sauce in each cap and steam. Put mushrooms under broiler and broil until the pesto is lightly browned.

- 3 tbs. commercial pesto
- ½ cup Silken (soft) light tofu
- ¼ cup reduced fat Monterey Jack cheese or part-skim mozzarella, grated and packed
- 3 to 4 cups cooked spaghetti noodles
- freshly shredded Parmesan cheese (optional)

1. In small food processor, blend pesto, tofu, and Monterey Jack or mozzarella cheese together until creamy and fairly smooth.
2. Place about half of the cooked noodles on each plate. Spread half the pesto cream sauce over the top of each serving of noodles. Microwave each on high power about 3 minutes, or until the pasta is nice and hot. Sprinkle parmesan cheese over the top if desired. Serve (makes two servings).

Per serving: 486 calories, 22 g protein, 72 g carbohydrate, 12 g fat, 3 g saturated fat, 11 mg cholesterol, 4 g fiber, 220 mg sodium. Calories from fat: 22%.
Vitamin A: 135 RE, Calcium: 248 mg, Folic Acid: 28 mcg.

 Breakfast Smoothie

- ½ cup soft, Silken style tofu, packed
- 1 banana, cut into 4 pieces
- 1 cup calcium-fortified, pulp-free orange juice
- ½ tsp. vanilla extract
- 5 ice cubes

Add all ingredients to a blender and whip at the highest setting for about 20 seconds or until the mixture is nice and frothy with no evidence of tofu. Pour into a tall glass and enjoy (makes one smoothie)!

Per serving: 285 calories, 8.5 g protein, 56 g carbohydrate, 4 g fat, 0 g saturated fat, 0 mg cholesterol, 2.5 g fiber, 26 mg sodium. Calories from fat: 12%.
Vitamin A: 20 RE, Calcium: 310 mg, Vitamin C: 106 mg, Folic Acid: 67 mcg.

Fruits in a flash

 ## Boysenberry-Banana Blast

The bananas and berries that are used in this fruit smoothie contribute all of the phytochemicals phenolic acids (if raspberries are used), catechins, and plant sterols that you need.

- ¾ cup frozen, unsweetened boysenberries or raspberries, partially thawed
- ½ cup lowfat boysenberry yogurt
- ½ banana, sliced
- ½ cup calcium-enriched cherry or grape juice

Add all ingredients to blender or food processor and purée until well blended, about 1 minute, and serve (makes one smoothie).

Per serving: 286 calories, 7 g protein, 64 g carbohydrate, 2 g fat, 5 mg cholesterol, 5 g fiber, 73 mg sodium, 275 mg calcium. Calories from fat: 6%.

 ## Strawberry Lemonade

The strawberries in this smoothie recipe contribute the phytochemicals phenolic acids and catechins, and the lemon juice in the lemonade may contribute some terpenes and carotenoids (which are found in citrus fruits).

- 1 cup frozen, unsweetened whole strawberries or ¾ cup sliced
- ½ cup prepared lemonade
- ½ cup lowfat lemon or plain yogurt

Add all ingredients to blender or food processor and purée until well blended, about 1 minute, and serve (makes one smoothie).

Per serving: 218 calories, 6.5 g protein, 46.5 g carbohydrate, 2 g fat, 5 mg cholesterol, 2.5 g fiber, 77 mg sodium, 210 mg calcium, 87 mg vitamin C. Calories from fat: 7 %.

 ## *Carrot Citrus Cooler*

- 4 ounces carrot juice
- 4 ounces calcium fortified orange tangerine (or orange) juice
- 4 ounces diet or regular 7-Up, Seltzer water, Club soda, or sparkling mineral water

Add all ingredients to tall drinking glass and stir. Add ice cubes if desired (makes one drink).

Per drink: 95 calories, 2 g protein, 21 g carbohydrate, 0 g fat, 0 saturated fat, 0 cholesterol, 1 g fiber, 92 mg sodium. Calories from fat: 0%.

Vitamin A: 350 % DV, Calcium: 20% DV, Vitamin C: 62% DV, Folic Acid: 8% DV.

 ## *Orange Sunrise*

- ½ cup calcium-fortified orange juice
- ½ cup reduced calorie (or regular) cranberry juice cocktail

Pour the orange juice into a clear drinking glass. Pour in the cranberry juice. Don't forget to watch the sunrise! (Makes one serving.)

Orange Juliet

- 1½ cups calcium-fortified orange juice
- ½ cup water
- ½ cup Egg Beaters egg substitute
- 1 tsp. vanilla extract
- 3 tbs. granulated sugar
- 1 heaping cup ice

Combine all of the ingredients in a blender set on the highest speed for exactly 1 minute. Pour into 2 glasses (makes 2 drinks).

Power vegetable recipes

Super Side Salad

This side salad is loaded with phytochemicals. The broccoli, tomatoes, and carrots, contributes the phytochemicals isothiocyanates, phenolic acids, terpenes, carotenoids, and plant sterols.

- 2 cups lettuce, shredded or chopped (fresh spinach leaves will add even more nutrients and phytochemicals)
- 3 cherry tomatoes
- ¼ cup canned kidney beans, drained and rinsed
- ¼ cup grated carrot
- ¼ cup raw chopped broccoli florets
- 3 tbs. reduced calorie Italian dressing (or similar)

1. Arrange lettuce in individual salad bowl or plate.

2.   Arrange tomatoes, beans, carrot, and broccoli over the top.

3.   Drizzle with your favorite reduced calorie dressing. Makes one serving (See salad dressing suggestions in Chapter 7).

Per serving: 151 calories, 5.5 g protein, 21 g carbohydrate, about 5 g fat, 0 g saturated fat, 3 mg cholesterol, 7.5 g fiber, 400 to 600 mg sodium. Calories from fat: about 29%.

Vitamin A: 1,176 RE, Calcium: 81 mg, Vitamin C: 74 mg, Vitamin E: 2.5 mg, Folic Acid: 223 mcg.

 Power Minestrone

This soup contains the phytochemicals phenolic acids, allyl sulfides, terpenes, 3-N-butyl phthalide, carotenoids and plant sterols. Make a batch and freeze individual servings in microwave-safe containers; they make a quick snack or side serving for a quick lunch or dinner.

- 5 cups low sodium beef broth (canned or from packet reconstituted with water)
- 3 carrots, diced
- 3 large celery stalks, sliced at a diagonal
- 1 onion, chopped
- 3 to 4 cloves garlic, minced or pressed
- 1 tsp. dried basil, crushed
- ½ tsp. dried oregano, crushed
- ¼ tsp. pepper
- 15-ounce can red kidney beans, drained and rinsed (or great northern beans)
- 15-ounce can stewed tomatoes
- 2 cups zucchini pieces (zucchini halved lengthwise and sliced)

- ½ cup tiny shell macaroni (or similar pasta)
- 4 tbs. freshly grated parmesan cheese (optional)

1. In a large saucepan combine broth, carrots, celery, onion, garlic, basil, oregano, and pepper. Bring to a boil; reduce heat. Cover; simmer for 15 minutes.
2. Stir in beans, tomatoes, zucchini, and macaroni. Return to a boil; cover and reduce heat to simmer. Cook 10 minutes more or until vegetables are tender.
3. Ladle into bowls; sprinkle parmesan cheese over the top of each, if desired (makes five large servings).

Per serving: 228 calories, 13.5 g protein, 38.5 g carbohydrate, 2 g fat, 0 g saturated fat, 0 mg cholesterol, 10.5 g fiber, 620 mg sodium (if using reduced-sodium beef broth). Calories from fat: 9%.

Vitamin A: 1287 RE, Calcium: 103 mg, Vitamin C: 27 mg, Vitamin E: 1 mg, Folic Acid: 87 mcg.

My favorite "fast" bean recipes

 ## Quick Microwave Bean Burrito

- ½ cup canned beans (your choice) drained and rinsed
- 2 tbs. nonfat or light sour cream
- 1 to 2 tbs. salsa
- 1 green onion, finely chopped
- 10-inch flour tortilla (burrito size)
- 1/3 cup (1 1/3 ounces) grated reduced fat Monterey Jack cheese

1. In a small bowl, blend the first four ingredients. Heat tortilla in the microwave for about 1 minute or until soft.
2. Sprinkle cheese over entire top of tortilla and spoon bean mixture evenly in center. Fold bottom end up, then roll up like a burrito. Microwave for an additional minute until burrito is heated throughout. Serve with salsa drizzled over the top, if desired.

Per burrito: 442 calories, 24 g protein, 61 g carbohydrate, 11 g fat, 4.5 g saturated fat, 20 mg cholesterol, 9 g fiber, 580 mg sodium. Calories from fat: 22%.
Vitamin A: 148 RE, Vitamin C: 12 mg, Vitamin E: 1.2 mg, Calcium: 422 mg, Folic Acid: 160 mcg.

 ## 3-Bean & Broccoli Salad

- 15-ounce can kidney beans, rinsed and drained
- 15-ounce can garbanzo beans, rinsed and drained
- 15-ounce can green beans or yellow wax beans, rinsed and drained
- ½ cup finely chopped onion
- 2 cups broccoli florets, slightly cooked in steamer or microwave
- $\frac{1}{3}$ cup of your favorite reduced fat or lite vinaigrette salad dressing (or mix one up yourself with 2 tbs. sherry or red wine vinegar, 1 1/2 tbs. olive oil, 3 tbs. apple juice and 1/2 packet of Good Seasons Garlic & Herb)

Add all the ingredients to a serving bowl and toss. Refrigerate until needed (makes about seven half-cup servings).

Per serving: 164 calories, 7.5 g protein, 28 g carbohydrate, 3 g fat, 0 g saturated fat, 0 mg cholesterol, 7.5 g fiber, 350 mg sodium. Calories from fat: 16 percent.
Vitamin A: 47 RE, Vitamin C: 28 mg, Vitamin E: 0.6 mg, Calcium: 53 mg, Folic Acid: 98 mcg.

 ## Salsa Bean Dip

- ¾ cups mild salsa (or your favorite salsa)
- ¼ cup diced onion
- 1 to 2 cloves garlic, crushed or minced
- ¾ cup canned black beans, drained and rinsed
- ¾ cup canned pinquitos or white beans, drained and rinsed
- ¼ cup fresh cilantro, coarsely chopped
- 1 tomato, chopped (optional)

Toss ingredients together in serving bowl. Refrigerate until needed. Serve with reduced fat tortilla chips, fresh flour tortillas, or quesidillas made with reduced fat cheese (makes five half-cup servings).

Per serving: 60 calories, 4 g protein, 9.5 g carbohydrate, 0.6 g fat, 0 saturated fat, 0 mg cholesterol, 5 g fiber, 450 mg sodium. Calories from fat: 9%.
Vitamin A: 70 RE, Vitamin C: 18 mg, Vitamin E: 0.4 mg, Calcium: 48 mg, Folic Acid: 35 mcg.

 _Chapter 6_

Navigating the Supermarket

Now that you have all those great recipes, you need to know how to navigate the supermarket. On the following pages, I will give you the best of what I have found in the way of taste, nutritional content, and what to look for when shopping.

Best-tasting soy products

I'll confess, I'm not one to normally seek out soy products. But I researched and taste-tested all the soy I could get my hands on. I never actually thought I would end up liking as many soy products as I did. The products I have listed I found in my neighborhood supermarket. You may have to go to your nearest natural foods store to find some of them.

Following are some of the best-tasting soy products I found. I have listed nutritional information as well.

Baked Tofu, 3-ounce serving

Baked Tofu (Soy Deli) Hickory flavor (several flavors are available)

140 calories, 18 g protein, 10 g carbohydrate, 3.5 grams fat, .5 g saturated fat, 0 mg cholesterol, 2 g fiber, 580 mg sodium, 10% DV calcium.

Tofu Burgers, 1 patty

Barbecue Tofu Burgers (Soy Deli) Tofu Burgers

210 calories, 15 g protein, 17 g carbohydrate, 9 g fat, 0 g saturated fat, 0 mg cholesterol, 1 g fiber, 200 mg sodium, 10% DV calcium.

Soy Milk, 1-cup serving

Silk Chocolate Dairyless Soy Beverage (WhiteWave, Inc.)

32 mg isoflavones, 108 calories, 5 g protein, 17 g carbohydrate, 2.5 g fat, 0 saturated fat, 0 cholesterol, 1 g fiber, 95 mg sodium, 30% DV calcium, 30% DV vitamin D, 50% DV vitamin B12.

"Silk" Dairyless Soy Beverage, unflavored (WhiteWave, Inc.)

35 mg isoflavones, 80 calories, 6 g protein, 9 g carbohydrate, 2.5 g fat, 0 saturated fat, 0 cholesterol, 0 fiber, 95 mg sodium, 30% DV calcium, 30% DV vitamin D, 50% DV vitamin B12.

Canned soybeans, half-cup serving

Westbrae Natural Organic Soy Beans

150 calories, 13 g protein, 11 g carbohydrate, 7 g fat, 1 g saturated fat, 0 mg cholesterol, 3 g fiber, 140 mg sodium, 10% DV calcium, 4% DV vitamin C.

Best bean bets

The following beans not only contain one of the phytoestrogens, but are also rich sources of several other important nutrients.

Soybeans, 1 cup cooked

175 mg calcium, phytoestrogens (lignans and isoflavones), 6 g fiber, 93 mcg folic acid, approximately 30 IU of vitamin E (100% DV).

Lentils, 1 cup cooked

38 mg calcium, lignans, 10 g fiber, 358 mcg folic acid.

Red Kidney beans, 1 cup cooked

50 mg calcium, phytoestrogens (lignans), 15 g fiber, 229 mcg folic acid.

Navy beans, 1 cup cooked

127 mg calcium, phytoestrogens (lignans), 16 g fiber, 255 mcg folic acid.

Pinto beans, 1 cup cooked

82 mg calcium, phytoestrogens (lignans), 19 g fiber, 294 mcg folic acid.

Canned bean soups and chili

Following are some canned bean side dishes or entrees that you could heat up during those busy weekday meals.

Tuscany-style Minestrone (Campbell's Home Cookin')

Per 1 cup: 190 calories, 5 g protein, 21 g carbohydrate, 9 g fat, 2 g saturated fat, 5 mg cholesterol, 5 g fiber, 870 mg sodium. Calories from fat: 42%. Vitamin A: 60% DV, Calcium: 8% DV, Vitamin C: 4% DV.

Lentil Classic Soup (Progresso)

Per cup: 140 calories, 9 g protein, 22 g carbohydrate, 2 g fat, 0 g saturated fat, 0 mg cholesterol, 7 g fiber, 750 mg sodium. Calories from fat: 13%.

Vitamin A: 15% DV, Calcium: 4% DV.

Savory Lentil (Campbell's Home Cookin')

Per cup: 130 calories, 8 g protein, 23 g carbohydrate, 1 g fat, 0 g saturated fat, 0 mg cholesterol, 4 g fiber, 770 mg sodium. Calories from fat: 7%.

Vitamin A: 60% DV, Calcium: 4% DV, Vitamin C: 2% DV.

Minestrone (Campbell's Healthy Request)

Per cup: 90 calories, 4 g protein, 17 g carbohydrate, 1 g fat, 0.5 g saturated fat, 0 mg cholesterol, 2 g fiber, 480 mg sodium. Calories from fat: 10%.

Vitamin A: 45% DV, Calcium: 2% DV.

Vegetarian Chili with Beans (Dennison's)

Per cup: 180 calories, 8 g protein, 35 g carbohydrate, 1 g fat, 0 g saturated fat, 0 mg cholesterol, 9 g fiber, 980 mg sodium. Calories from fat: 5%.

Vitamin A: 25% DV, Calcium: 10% DV.

Vegetarian Chili with Beans (Hormel)

Per cup: 200 calories, 12 g protein, 38 g carbohydrate, 1 g fat, 0 g saturated fat, 0 mg cholesterol, 7 g fiber, 780 mg sodium. Calories from fat: 5%.

Vitamin A: 25% DV, Calcium: 6% DV.

Ranch House Chicken Chili with Beans (Stagg)

Per cup: 290 calories, 19 g protein, 32 g carbohydrate, 9 g fat, 3 g saturated fat, 50 mg cholesterol, 6 g fiber, 810 mg sodium. Calories from fat: 28%.
Vitamin A: 10% DV, Calcium: 6% DV.

Best produce picks

Fruits and vegetables are a bounty of important nutrients. Depending on the fruits and vegetables, many are sources of the following:

- phytoestrogens (lignans and isoflavones).
- other phytochemicals, besides phytoestrogens.
- the mineral boron, helpful toward improving estrogen levels after menopause and decreasing calcium loss at any age.
- calcium (dark green leafy vegetables).
- antioxidants (vitamin C, beta carotene) and the powerful micronutrient, folic acid.
- fiber.

Check the table on the next page to see which fruits and vegetables are rich in which nutrients.

Antioxidant power houses

The following fruits contain 100 percent or more of the daily value (recommended amount) for beta-carotene (Beta) or vitamin C (C):

- cantaloupe, 1 cup (C)
- Guava, half (C)
- kiwi, 1 (C)

- mango, 1 (Beta, C)
- orange, 1 (C)
- papaya, half (C)

Fruits rich in phytoestrogens

Lignans	Isoflavones	Boron
	apples	apples
		apricots
		avocados
		bananas
	berries	
		blueberries
		cantaloupe
		cherries (sour)
	citrus fruits	
		currants: red/black
		figs
		gooseberries
		grapefruit
	grapes	grapes
		mandarin oranges
		mangoes
		papaya
		peaches
pears		pears
		persimmons (American)
plums		plums
		quinces
		red raspberries
	strawberries	strawberries

The following vegetables contain 100 percent or more of the daily value (recommended amount) for beta-carotene (Beta) or vitamin C (C):

- beet greens, 1 cup boiled (C)
- bell pepper, red or yellow, half (C)

- broccoflower, 1 cup steamed (C)
- broccoli, 1 cup cooked (C)
- Brussels sprouts, 1 cup cooked (C)
- butternut squash, ½ cup baked, mashed (Beta)
- carrot, 1 (Beta)
- carrot slices, ½ cup steamed (Beta)
- cauliflower, 1 cup boiled (C)
- chili peppers, ¼ cup canned or raw (C)
- Chinese cabbage, 1 cup steamed (C)
- dandelion greens, 1 cup boiled (Beta)
- dock/sorrel greens, 1 cup raw chopped (C)
- green pea pods, 1 cup cooked (C)
- hubbard squash, 1 cup baked cubes (Beta)
- kale, 1 cup boiled (Beta, C)
- kohlrabi, 1 cup boiled (C)
- lamb's quarters, ½ cup boiled (Beta)
- peas, 1 cup raw (C)
- pumpkin, ½ cup boiled or canned (Beta)
- snow peas, 1 cup steamed (C)
- spinach, 1 cup boiled (Beta)
- sweet potato, 1 baked without skin or ½ cup canned (Beta)
- turnip greens, 1 cup boiled (Beta)
- yams, orange, ½ cup mashed (Beta)
- Calcium-rich vegetables
- collard greens, boiled, 1 cup (350 mg)
- turnip greens, boiled, 1 cup (250 mg)
- spinach, boiled, 1 cup (280 mg)
- black-eyed peas, boiled, 1 cup (210 mg)
- dandelion greens, cooked, 1 cup (150 mg)
- broccoli, cooked, 1 cup (95 mg)

- kale, boiled, ½ cup (90 mg)
- boy choy, boiled, ½ cup (80 mg)

Vegetables rich in phytoestrogens

Lignans	Isoflavones	Boron
		alfalfa sprouts
asparagus		asparagus
beets		beets
broccoli	broccoli	broccoli
	cabbage	cabbage
carrot	carrot	carrot
cauliflower		cauliflower
		celery root
		Chinese cabbage
		corn
	cucumbers	cucumbers
		dandelion greens
	eggplant	
		endive
garlic	garlic	
green peppers	green peppers	
iceberg lettuce		
leeks		
	lettuce (all types)	lettuce
onions		onions
	parsley	
	peppers (all types)	peppers
		radishes
rutabaga (roots/stems)		
snow peas		
	soybeans	soybeans
		spinach
squash	squash	
sweet potatoes		sweet potatoes
	tomatoes	tomatoes
turnips		turnips
	yams	

Fatty Acid Do's and Don'ts

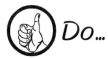 *Do...*

...buy 100-percent canola oil as your vegetable oil. It can be used in stir-frying, sautéing, and baking.

...buy 100-percent canola margarine with the first ingredient being "liquid canola oil." Use it as a spread and in some cooking and baking. If it contains approximately 11 grams fat per tablespoon, it should work well where butter or regular margarine are called for.

...buy extra virgin olive oil. You can use it in cold salads and dressings and for medium temperature sautéing and simmering. It can't be used in higher temperature frying, though.

...buy canola or olive oil cooking spray or use canola or olive oil in your refillable oil sprayers.

...buy canola-based salad dressings, many of which also happen to be lower in fat and calories. To reduce calories of regular dressings, blend one-half cup dressing with one-half cup fruit juice or nonalcoholic wine or champagne (or lowfat milk for a creamy dressing).

...buy canola-based mayonnaise whenever possible. To make a great-tasting mayonnaise mixture, blend mayonnaise with fat-free or light sour cream.

...eat fish two times a week to increase your fish source of omega-3 fatty acids. The best known fish sources of omega-3 fatty acids are sardines, herring, anchovies, whitefish and bluefish, salmon, and mackerel. Fair fish sources are swordfish, canned tuna, rainbow trout, striped bass, pacific oysters, and squid.

...eat more canola, soybeans and soybean products, spinach, mustard greens, walnuts, and flaxseed, to get the plant sources of alpha-linolenic acid.

...buy the best-tasting lower fat options in processed food categories that are normally high in trans fatty acids (chips, crackers, cookies, and other commercial baked goods).

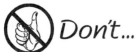 *Don't...*

...buy margarine that lists "partially hydrogenated" or "hydrogenated" oils as the first ingredient. These margarines will most likely contain a high amount of trans fatty acids.

...use a lot of high omega-6 vegetable oils in your homecooking, such as corn, safflower, and sunflower oil.

...buy high fat processed foods that use partially hydrogenated oils, such as chips, crackers, cookies, and other high-fat baked goods, on a regular basis.

4 brands of 100% pure canola oil

Canola oil has a nice, neutral flavor that won't interfere with the other flavors in the dish or baked product. When a neutral tasting oil is needed, I call on canola. I found these brands of 100-percent canola oil in my supermarket:

- Mazola canola oil.
- Pure Wesson canola oil.
- Smart Beat canola oil.
- Safeway 100-percent pure canola oil.

4 monounsaturated fat-rich salad dressings

There were many other salad dressings that did list canola oil or olive oil in its list of ingredients, but they also listed another oil (such as soy oil). When it is an "either-or" situation, you can't be sure the bottle you are buying contains canola or olive oil. So, I only listed the salad dressings that exclusively used canola or olive oil.

$^{1}/_{3}$ Less Fat Red Wine Vinaigrette (Seven Seas)
(contains canola oil)
Per 2 tablespoons: 45 calories, 4 g fat
Italian Reduced Fat Dressing (Kraft)
(Contains canola oil)
Per 2 tablespoons: 50 calories, 4.5 g fat
Olive Oil Vinaigrette (Wishbone)
(Contains olive oil)
Per 2 tablespoons: 60 calories, 5 g fat
Balsamic Italian (Bernstein's)
(Contains canola oil)
Per 2 tablespoons: 110 calories, 11 g fat

How to read a margarine label

Margarine labels today can be very confusing. But right away we can rule out stick margarine labels. Because stick margarine needs to be extremely solid (to maintain a stick form) it will contain hydrogenated oil as the first ingredient—which means it will contain mostly saturated fat and trans fatty acids.

So let's talk about tub margarine. These are more likely to have liquid canola oil, olive oil, or soybean oil as the first ingredient. They will have the highest monounsaturated fats and the lowest saturated fat. The tricky part comes when you want to know how much trans fatty acids your tub margarine contains. Manufacturers do not yet have to list the grams of trans fatty acids—just saturated fat. Most of the manufacturers also list the grams of polyunsaturated fat and monounsaturated fat.

So you can play detective and figure out how many grams of trans fatty acid your tub margarine contains by process of elimination. Take the total amount of fat grams and subtract the grams of saturated fat, poly- and monounsaturated; what is left is the grams of trans fatty acid. If your tub margarine contain no more than 2 grams of trans fatty acids per tablespoon, you have found a pretty good margarine!

What about butter?

Because eating a moderate lowfat diet is good advice for most of us, indiscriminate use of butter (and margarine, for that matter) is still a nutritional no-no. Butter contains the same amount of fat per tablespoon as stick margarine (and even some tub margarine) and it contains 7 grams saturated fat per tablespoon while delivering 3.5 grams monounsaturated and 0.5 gram polyunsaturated fat. It does contain a little cholesterol (10 milligrams per teaspoon serving), where margarine doesn't have any.

So the question really is: "How much butter are we talking about?" Are you using a teaspoon here and a teaspoon there or do you glob it on? If you are a relentless globber, you are better off with one of the tub margarines. But if you can take butter "lightly," there may still be a place for butter in your kitchen.

Are you going nuts?

Nuts have gotten a bad nutritional rap in the past because they are, lets face it, high in fat grams and calories. But new research is portraying nuts as "wholesome" food (contributing fiber and other helpful nutrients) and the nuts high in monounsaturated fats and/or omega-3 fatty acids are particularly good to eat. What about the fat grams and calories? Exercise the "M" word: Moderation. One-eighth cup serving of nuts goes a long way when you mix it with dried fruit, cereal, or blend it in a muffin or stir-fry. Of course you can eat a handful right out of the bag. Depending on the size of your hand, a handful could be just the right portion of nuts. The trick is keeping your hand out of the bag after one or two reaches.

Nuts rich in mostly monounsaturated fats:

- $1/_8$ cup macadamia nuts contain 9.4 g monounsaturated fat (78% of total fat)
- $1/_8$ cup hazelnuts contain 8 g monounsaturated fat (85% of total fat)
- $1/_8$ cup whole almonds contain 5.8 g monounsaturated fat (65% of total fat)
- $1/_8$ cup pecan halves contain 5.5 g monounsaturated fat (63% of total fat)
- $1/_8$ cup pistachio nuts contain 5.2 g monounsaturated fat (60% of total fat)

Just the flax, please

Once you've found a health food store that carries flaxseed, that's half the battle. The rest is knowing which form of flaxseed to buy and how to use and store it.

Once you grind the seeds (and you'll want to, because the body enzymes can get to the beneficial chemicals better this way), it is highly perishable (lasting only 30 days if refrigerated). Flaxseed oil, too, will keep for only 30 days refrigerated. You can't cook or bake with it (heat makes it rancid) and the oil doesn't contain the beneficial lignans and fiber (found in the ground flaxseed) because when making the oil, they are both removed in the process.

Because we want *all* of the benefits from flaxseed, I recommend buying whole or ground flaxseeds not flaxseed oil. You will find the seeds (often in bulk bins) in health food stores. You might even be able to find a product called "Fortified Flax" which is a preground flaxseed (that looks like cornmeal). It is fortified with nutrients, such as vitamins C and E, to stabilize it against oxidation which keeps it from going rancid. Once a package of preground flaxseed is opened, keep it refrigerated. Whatever you don't use in 6 months, throw away.

 <u>Chapter 7</u>

Restaurant Rules to Live By

I don't know about you but I love eating out in restaurants. And often when Americans are eating "in" they are, in actuality, eating "out"—take-out has never been more popular.

The problem with restaurant hopping is that you don't know what you're getting in terms of calories, fat grams, saturated fat, and the like. It's not like a supermarket where almost everything has a nutrition information label and ingredient list. Even fast-food chains have the nutrition information available in a pamphlet or via a toll-free number. That's not the case with restaurants.

Even if I told you what the nutrition content was for something like fettuccini alfredo, chow mein, or meatloaf and mashed potatoes, every chef in every restaurant is going to use a different recipe. And every chef is going to go lighter or heavier on the butter, oil, or cream. On the bright side, you can ask for something to be served or prepared a certain way, and it usually isn't a problem.

Then there are the "restaurant chains," those restaurants that are midway between the fast-food chains and fancy restaurants: Applebee's, Chili's, or Red Robin, and the like. It's the type of place where every member of the family can be happy. The kids can have a burger while the adults can have grilled chicken salad, pasta, steak, or fish. Everybody's happy.

True, you can stumble upon absolutely loads of saturated fat and calories at these places, but you also have many healthful choices, too. Most offer salads with low-calorie dressing, baked potatoes, grilled chicken, and fish. Several chains even have "lite" or "healthful" sections on their menus.

To help keep the right nutrients high and the wrong nutrients low, here are some tips to take with you when you are out and about.

Ask for what you want

Remember the phrase, "The customer is always right"? Well, if you would like your dish prepared a certain way, ask. More often than not, they will do it for you because they want you to come back. Here are some things you can ask for that will help you meet the 10 Food Steps to Freedom.

- **Add tofu** to any dish you want to order from a Chinese restaurant.
- **Add tofu** as an extra ingredient to your favorite burrito.
- **Substitute a baked potato or in season vegetables** for the french fries that normally come with your entrée or sandwich.
- **Cut the cream.** Ask for your burger, fish or chicken sandwich to be prepared without the mayonnaise, tartar sauce, or "special sauce." If they don't take it off, wipe it off.

- **Hold the mayo.** Order your sandwich with ketchup or mustard instead of mayonnaise.
- **Ask for half as much sauces** with your pasta or meat dishes. High fat sauces should be the garnish, not a large portion of the meal.
- **Sauté in wine, not butter.** If there is a dish you really want to try, but it says that it is sautéed or simmered in cream or butter, ask that it be simmered in wine or broth instead.
- **Ask for the dressing on the side** so you decide how much is used.
- **Ask for grilled chicken** instead of fried for chicken salads and sandwiches.
- **Ask that the skin be removed** from your chicken before it is prepared.
- **Switch sauces.** If you want to order manicotti, cannelloni, chicken, or fish, and it comes with a creamy, butter-laden sauce, switch to a better sauce. Ask for marinara, marsala, or a wine sauce.

General rules

Watch out for anything described as "creamy," "breaded," "crispy," or "fried." That's not to say that you shouldn't have these at all, but these items traditionally score very high on the calorie, fat, saturated fat, and trans fatty acid meters and it isn't healthwise to order them often.

- **Just grill it!** Grilled chicken and fish are two of the healthiest things you can possibly order at restaurants.
- **Go for the greens.** Vegetables always seem to taste better in restaurants. Make a point to enjoy them. And ask that the chef skip the butter when the vegetables are cooked.

- **Enjoy salads.** Side and dinner salads are great, just remember to order the dressing on the side.

- **Hold the bacon, cheese, and mayo.** Those grilled chicken sandwiches (and even the quarter-pound burgers for that matter) are a great choice until we start dressing them up with all the trimmings: bacon, cheese, mayonnaise, etc. Add mustard, ketchup, or barbecue sauce instead, skip the cheese, load up on lettuce and tomato, and leave the bacon for breakfast.

- **Order lean mean meats.** Sirloin steak and filet mignon are two of your best steak bets, especially if you are in the habit of trimming off any visible fat.

Sandwich strategies

Some sandwiches rate better on the nutrition meter than others. You decide how healthy you want your sandwich to be. Three steps follow.

1. *Select the better fillers:* roast chicken or turkey breast, and roast beef are great choices; a lean ham will also do well. Chicken, shrimp, and tuna salad from a deli often are completely drenched in mayonnaise. You can make light versions at home, but when ordering out, I would choose a lean meat instead.

2. *Dress your sandwich wisely.* A safe choice is mustard. Italian delicatessens will sometimes lightly wet the bread with an olive oil mixture, which will at least add the more desirable monounsaturated fat. If you absolutely must have mayonnaise, have it spread on lightly.

3. *Choose your best bread.* Whole wheat breads will contribute fiber and micronutrients. French rolls, whole wheat sliced bread, or even bagels are okay. Just avoid croissants!

Great takeout choices

When you're in a rush, sometimes the easiest way to eat is to do take out. We have lots of options out there: Chinese, burrito shops, BBQ takeout, pizza parlors, and sandwich shops.

Pizza

One large slice of thin-crust tomato pizza with a large green salad with Italian dressing, or a bowl of soup.

Even better: Top your pizza or salad with whatever veggies you wish.

[565 calories, 19 g fat, 4 g saturated fat. Calories from fat: 29%.]

Chinese Stir-fry

Shrimp and vegetable stir-fry with steamed rice.

Even better: Don't toss the fortune cookie—it's only 30 fat-free calories!

[606 calories, 14 g fat, 3 g saturated fat. Calories from fat: 21%.]

Rotisserie

Enjoy the turkey breast with new potatoes, steamed vegetables, and hot cinnamon apples.

[595 calories, 9 g fat, 2 g saturated fat. Calories from fat: 14%.]

Vegetable Burrito

With black beans or whole pintos and rice on a whole wheat tortilla.

Even better: Add tofu to your vegetable burrito, and ask for whole beans, if they give you a choice.

[500 calories (approximately), 9 g fat, 1 g saturated fat. Calories from fat: 14 to 20%.]

Best choices...

If you are at a deli

Roast chicken or turkey breast or roast beef on a French roll or whole wheat bread with mustard, lettuce, and tomato.

If you are at a Chinese restaurant

Enjoy the dishes that aren't breaded and deep fried and partner them up with some steamed rice. This is also a great opportunity to include lots of vegetables and tofu. Here are some suggestions:

- Vegetable/tofu chow mein
- Tofu with vegetables
- Curry tofu
- Chicken with broccoli or snow peas
- Shrimp in black bean sauce

If you are at a Japanese restaurant

Start off your meal with phytoestrogen-rich miso soup. Then enjoy the salmon teriyaki and get your allotment of omega-3 fatty acids. Or try some vegetable sushi.

If you are at a French bistro

The key to eating French food is: *Watch your sauces.* You may start off well with a lean chicken breast or fish fillet, but it may end up doused in hollandaise or béarnaise sauce (at 450 calories, most of which are from fat) per half cup. You are better off with béchamel sauce, which has 228 calories per half cup, or Bordelaise sauce (wine sauce) with 155 calories per half cup. Other good choices are:

- Steamed mussels.
- Fish poached in wine.

If you are at an Italian restaurant

Anything with marinara will probably be all right. Marinara sauce is traditionally low in fat and high in flavor. And as a bonus, there are phytochemicals in the tomatoes that are actually more active after cooking. Marsala sauce is also a good choice because it is made with wine.

Pesto sauce is going to be high in fat, but usually olive oil is the fat used (high in monounsaturated fat). Pesto sauce is so rich in flavor that a little goes a long way, so ask for half as much pesto on your pasta.

If you are at a rotisserie restaurant

Pass up the chicken pot pie. If you go for the roasted chicken, skip the skin. Pass up the creamed spinach, and ask for the baked new potatoes, baked sweet potatoes, or fresh fruit. Opt for the meat loaf sandwich (no cheese), chicken soup with corn bread and zucchini marsala.

If you are at a Mexican restaurant

Soft tortillas are better than "crispy" because the crispy are deep fried. Burritos are better than chimichangas because the chimichangas are deep fried. The Spanish rice is traditionally low in fat and helps round out your Mexican meal. If you have the choice between refried beans and whole beans, go for the whole, but both with give you a serving of beans and a boost of fiber and that's a good thing. Enjoy the guacamole (high in monounsaturated fat) and sour cream but try to keep it to a tablespoon or two (the calories will start to add up.) A tablespoon garnish of each will only add about 100 calories. Try:

- veggie burritos.
- bean burritos (add rice if you can to help "fill" you up).
- chicken soft tacos with lettuce, tomatoes, salsa, rice and whole beans.
- chicken enchiladas (easy on the extra cheese or sour cream).

- chicken fajitas, shrimp or vegetable fajitas (if you've got to opt for the steak fajitas, go easy on the cheese and/or sour cream; the avocado is high in favorable monounsaturated fat).

- chicken tamales. Although traditionally made with lard, they are usually pretty low in calories (around 300 calories for two small tamales). Technically you could add some rice and beans and make a balanced meal.

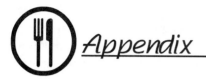

2 Menopause Makeovers

eading about what and how you need to eat is one thing. Doing it is quite another. Let me walk you through two nutrition makeovers—one is a 45-year-old thin woman approaching perimenopause concerned about osteoporosis and keeping her energy high. The other is a 55-year-old, almost postmenopausal woman, still battling weight gain and several perimenopausal symptoms.

Let's take a look at a typical day of food and drink for both these women and then help them incorporate the 10 Food Steps to Freedom.

Eating for energy and strong bones

Lori is a busy 45-year-old mother of two, juggling career and kids. She works at home in Florida as a computer software consultant. Her nutrition goal is to eat for high energy. Lori gets so busy she often forgets to eat and has to force herself to plan meals and snacks just to maintain her weight. She finds that she sometimes has "low energy moments"—which she desperately wants to avoid in the future. Because of her petite frame, ethnic background, and family history, she is most concerned about preventing osteoporosis.

Vital statistics

Height: 5'6"
Weight: 120 pounds
Marital and mother status: divorced mother of two

Tuesday

7 a.m.	2 cappuccinos (4 oz. espresso + 4 oz. 1% lowfat milk)
	1 slice whole wheat toast with 1 tbs. all-fruit jam
9 a.m.	instant coffee with 4 oz. 1% lowfat milk
	1/4 nectarine
	1 container lowfat peach yogurt (6 oz.)
10 a.m.	6 oz. orange juice
Noon	1 apple + 3 tbs. creamy peanut butter
	1 "lite" turkey hot dog with bun
	1/2 oz. potato chips
	6 oz. orange juice
4 p.m.	1 cup Honey Nut Cheerios
7 p.m.	1 beer (12 oz.)
	1 cup white rice + 1 cup seasoned black beans
	(sautéed with olive oil, garlic, onion, ginger)
	1 small mixed green salad
	(with olive oil and vinegar dressing)
	1 small slice watermelon
	1 "sliver" key lime pie with graham cracker crust
	2 mini peanut butter cups

Note: Lori drank about 4 cups of water throughout the day.

Exercise habits

Besides "running around" with her kids, Lori exercises at a gym twice a week (30 minutes on a treadmill and 20 minutes of strength training with weights).

Nutrition analysis

Calories	2,207 (108% RDA)
Protein	68 g (156% RDA) (12% total calories)
Carbohydrates	316 g (57% of total calories)
Fat	74 g (30% of total calories)
Saturated fat	18.5 g (7.5% of total calories)
Monounsaturated fat	32 g (13% of total calories)
Cholesterol	32 mg
Vitamin A (total)	1,175 RE (147% RDA)
Vitamin B1	1.6 mg (161% RDA)
Vitamin B2	2.2 mg (179% RDA)
Vitamin B3	22 mg (166% RDA)
Vitamin B6	1.7 mg (109% RDA)
Vitamin B12	4 mcg (201% RDA)
Folic acid	386 mcg (some researchers suggest 400 mcg per day)
Vitamin C	199 mg (332% RDA) (some researchers are now recommending 500 mg per day for the heart)
Vitamin E	7 mg (88% RDA) (some researchers are recommending 400 IU per day for heart disease prevention and increased immune function)
Calcium	1,076 mg (new recommendations on "optimal daily calcium" are 1000 mg for women between ages 25 and 50)
Iron	17.5 mg (117% RDA)
Magnesium	376 mg (134% RDA) (some researchers recommend 240 mg per day for the heart and bones)
Selenium	56.7 mcg (103% RDA) (some researchers recommend 200 mcg for the heart; selenium is an antioxidant)
Sodium	1,989 mg (it is a good idea to consume no more than 3000 mg a day)
Zinc	8 mg (66% RDA)

What is she doing right?

Lori is into a nice habit of eating small meals through the day (Food Step #6). Particularly in the morning hours, Lori has a meal or snack every couple of hours. As her day goes on, though, and her parental responsibilities kick in, the space between her meals/snacks widens.

Lori avoids high fat and high sugar foods, for the most part, while still letting herself enjoy reasonable amounts of dessert-type foods, such as her mini peanut butter cups and small slice of key lime pie (Food Step #8).

Lori eats beans often (Food Step #3) probably because she lives in Florida where many restaurants and food stops offer delicious bean fare.

Lori wants energy and she scores really well with the micronutrients that assist in making energy. For example, Lori got more than 100 percent of the RDA for all the B vitamins.

Given Lori's petite size and ethnicity, she is at higher risk of developing osteoporosis later in life. This is another good reason to cut the caffeine down a bit. Her calcium intake, though, meets the new recommendations and her magnesium intake is also high (magnesium helps bones, too). Her yogurt and lowfat milk came to her rescue here (Food Step 7).

Lori has switched to using canola and olive oil, both high in monounsaturated fats, and she has a fairly favorable fatty acid profile in her nutrition analysis—her saturated fat was nice and low, while her monounsaturated fat was the highest of the three (saturated, mono and polyunsaturated fats)—Food Step #4.

What can she improve upon?

Lori depends on her caffeine rush to get her through her morning hours. She may be experiencing her "low energy moments" due to the energy let down from the caffeine. For such a small body, she is pumping in quite a bit of caffeine (8 ounces of straight espresso and a cup of regular coffee a day). The high amounts of caffeine could be robbing some of the calcium her body so desperately needs to hold onto. If she could gradually cut down to one cup of caffeinated coffee per morning, she would be on her way to meeting Food Step #5.

Lori does a great job of getting her fruit servings in, but needs a boost in the vegetable department. Having some vegetable snacks around may help and making sure she has a vegetable with her lunch meal would also help (Food Step #2).

Lori should consider a nicely balanced multivitamin with minerals to help meet her requirements for zinc and the higher suggested intake for folic acid. When she starts eating more vegetables, her folic acid intake will improve too. Probably most important, though, is her very low intake of vitamin E. Many researchers are recommending 400 IU supplements a day for several reasons (higher immune function, antioxidant benefits, and other heart disease prevention benefits). Lori currently only gets 7 IU of vitamin E.

Lori could add a couple teaspoons of ground flaxseed to her daily orange juice (Food Step #9). Because she has never tried flaxseed she will need to start slowly, adding 1/4 teaspoon and working up to the tablespoon slowly, unless an allergic reaction is noticed.

Lori doesn't like tofu, therefore Food Step #1 gets a bit more challenging. She does, however, eat beans often. She might try adding canned organic soybeans (available in some markets) to some her favorite bean dishes. Lori also enjoys cafe lattes (soon to be mostly decaf). So she could try using fresh chocolate soy milk to make iced and hot lattes.

In hot flash hell

Alice is 55 and lives in Northern California. She entered perimenopause with a bang at the age of 50. She noticed frequent hot flashes, occasional insomnia, and looking back, this is when she began losing the battle of the bulge. She is now managing her hot flashes (and several other perimenopause symptoms) naturally by avoiding wine and spicy foods (hot flash triggers) and supplementing her daily diet with a couple servings of soy.

She has always struggled with a little extra weight and perimenopause is no exception. Her goals are to get through the remainder of perimenopause as comfortably as possible and to keep extra weight to a minimum. Because she mostly eats vegetarian meals (eating beans almost every day), Alice is worried she isn't getting all the nutrients she needs. She doesn't eat red meat and tries to have fish a couple times a week. The one food Alice craves on an almost daily basis is chocolate. And she tends to have her "sweet" cravings in the afternoon.

Vital statistics

Height: 5'3"

Weight: 160 pounds

Marital Status: married

Occupation: Recently retired, has started a small home-based business

Monday

6 a.m.	6 oz. coffee mixed with 6 oz. chocolate soy milk
	* went on a 3 mile walk (1 hour)
8 a.m.	1 1/2 cups Cheerios
	1 1/2 tablespoons oat bran
	1/2 banana, sliced
	1/2 cup nonfat milk

1 cup calcium fortified orange juice
* took vitamins: 1 Centrum Silver
                 1,000 mg calcium tablets
                 1,000 mg vitamin C
                 400 IU vitamin E

9:30 a.m.   handful of peanuts

11:30 a.m.   2 slices whole wheat bread
3 ounces baked tofu
1/2 cup bean salad (carrots, red pepper, green beans, kidney beans, dressed with a reduced-fat vinaigrette with olive oil)

3 p.m.   4 Triscuit crackers
1 slice of reduced-fat cheese
1 tangerine

6:30 p.m.   chicken with rice casserole
(1 skinless chicken breast, 3/4 cup steamed rice, 1/4 cup peas, apricot fruit jam blended with honey mustard for a sauce)
1/2 cup acorn squash, baked, dressed with 1/2 teaspoon butter + a sprinkle of brown sugar
1 slice French bread (no butter)
1 cup salad (iceberg lettuce, carrots, avocado, garbanzo beans dressed with fat-free Italian dressing)

8 p.m.   2 cups herb tea (decaf)
1 sliver mocha chocolate cake (1/4 of regular slice)

9 p.m.   2 tablespoons chocolate chips

Note: Alice drank about 5 tall glasses of water throughout the day.

Exercise habits

Alice goes on a 3 mile walk (1 hour) with her two golden retrievers (and 2 walking buddies) 6 times a week. She also attends a yoga class 2 times a week.

Nutrition analysis

Calories	2,075 (98% RDA)
Protein	97 g (166% RDA) (18% of total calories)
Carbohydrates	323 g (59% of total calories)

Fat	56 g (23% of total calories)
Saturated fat	16 g (7% of total calories)
Monounsaturated fat	21 g (9% of total calories)
Cholesterol	105 mg
Vitamin A (total)	1,554 RE (194% RDA)
Vitamin B1	2.6 mg (246% RDA)
Vitamin B2	1.9 mg (148% RDA)
Vitamin B3	35 mg (252% RDA)
Vitamin B6	2.9 mg (180% RDA)
Vitamin B12	2.9 mg (143% RDA)
Folic acid	397 mcg (some researchers suggest 400 mcg per day)
Vitamin C	233 mg (388% RDA) (some researchers are now recommending 500 mg per day for the heart)
Vitamin E	6.3 mg (78% RDA) (some researchers are recommending 400 IU per day for heart disease prevention and increased immune function)
Calcium	990 mg (new recommendation on "optimal daily calcium" is 500 mg for women over 50 not on HRT)
Iron	29 mg (290% RDA)
Magnesium	531 mg (190% RDA) (some researchers recommend 240 mg per day for the heart and bones)
Selenium	104 mcg (190% RDA) (some researchers recommend 200 mcg for the heart; selenium is an antioxidant, too)
Sodium	2,134 mg (it is a good idea to consume no more than 3000 mg a day)
Zinc	10.5 mg (88% RDA)

What is she doing right?

Alice has the first three food steps all sewn up. She eats tofu or soy milk almost every day, she ate about five servings of fruits and vegetables this particular day, and she eats a serving of beans almost every day. This is probably easier for her than it would be for most women, just because she is a self described "part-time vegetarian."

Alice definitely chooses her beverages wisely, drinking a good amount of water through the day. She has cut back to just the one cup of caffeinated coffee she needs to jump start her morning and rarely drinks soda and alcohol. She has a glass of nonfat milk, a cup of calcium-fortified orange juice, and a cup of calcium-rich soy milk almost every day, which helps her meet Food Step #7 and her high calcium requirements.

Alice is definitely minimizing extra calories by avoiding high fat and high sugar foods (Food Step #8). Her total calorie intake was within normal limits, with 23 percent of the calories coming from fat. She does crave chocolate, though, and lets herself have a little almost every day—preventing feelings of deprivation and the impulse to overeat.

Alice does a pretty good job of eating small frequent meals through the day and eating light at night. She might feel better with a more substantial snack in the afternoon, though.

What can she improve upon?

Alice might want to switch from orange juice to other beneficial juices (grapefruit, carrot, purple grape juice) from time to time—just to make life more interesting. Alice could stand to add a fruit or two into her snacking repertoire. She had about 1 1/2 fruit servings not including her orange juice.

Alice has drastically cut down on fats just to help her and her husband in their weight loss efforts, but I think she could improve her monounsaturated fat intake by using some olive or canola oil in salad dressings (instead of the less satisfying fat-free versions they use). They haven't been buttering their bread to reduce fat and saturated fat, but they might want to try a good canola oil tub margarine that contains almost no trans fatty acids and saturated fats and mostly monounsaturated fats (because the first ingredient is liquid canola oil).

Alice is religious about her daily vitamin supplements and has selected a great multivitamin with minerals for her needs and takes an appropriate amount of vitamin E. She probably doesn't need quite as much calcium as she is currently taking (1,000 mg). She is getting a good amount from her food choices, 1,000 milligrams, not to mention the calcium in her multivitamin, 200 milligrams. She could definitely cut down to one 500-milligram tablet. If she continues to take two tablets, though, she should take one in the morning and one later in the day.

Alice should consider sprinkling a couple teaspoons of ground flaxseed in her daily salad or juice. She could use the added omega-3 fatty acids in flaxseed; the phytoestrogens and cancer prevention properties couldn't hurt either. Doing whatever she can to prevent cancer is a priority for Alice. She knows that being overweight increases her risk.

Exercise is Alice's middle name, what with the almost daily three-mile dog walks. But Alice admits only part of her 60-minute walk is at a fast walking pace. She might notice more body fat loss if she were to have closer to 60 minutes of powerwalking, several times a week. Her yoga class is indeed increasing her flexibility and muscle strength, but Alice might consider some additional strength training to help combat the natural decline in muscle mass as we age and to help increase her metabolic rate (which could help with the weight loss efforts).

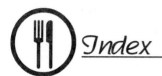 _Index_

starting age, 10-11
surgical, 11
Minimizing calories, 92-94
Monounsaturated fat, 21, 50, 66-67
Moodiness, 15, 43-44
  battling, 44-45

Nausea, battling, 43, 49
Night sweats, 27, 33-34
North American Menopause Society, 14, 24
  address, 25
Nuts, 132-133

Omega-3 fatty acids, 21, 50, 52, 61, 64-66, 68, 129
Omega-6 fatty acids, 50, 65, 68-69
Omega-9 fatty acids, 66
Osteoporosis
  and HRT, 16-19, 22-23
  and postmenopause, 21
  defined, 23
  increased risk of, 11
  reducing risk with foods, 53-55
  risk factors, 24
  tests, 23
Ovaries, removal of, 11
Ovulation, defined, 10

Perimenopause, 9, 11
  and HRT, 16-19
  defined, 10

first signs of, 12
number one complaint about, 12
top 10 symptoms, 27-46
Period
  changes in, 12
  first, and relationship to menopause, 11
Phytoestrogens, 28, 37-38, 61, 75-76
  foods rich in, 30
Polyunsaturated fat, 68
Postmenopause, 20-21
Practitioner, questions to ask, 9-25
Pregnancy, 13, 14-15
Premenstrual syndrome (PMS) 12, 15
Produce, best picks, 125-128
Progesterone, 15, 16
Progestin, 15, 16
Progestogen, 14

Questions, writing down, 9

Recipes, 101-120
Restaurant rules, 135-142

Saturated fat, 50, 67
Sexual activity, increased, 36-38
Sexually transmitted diseases, 20
Smoking, 11
  and blood lipids, 21